A.I.D.S.
Facts

Mr. Robert K. Boscarato

A.I.D.S. Facts

DEDICATION

Insert dedication text here. Insert dedication text here. Insert dedication text here. Insert dedication text here. Insert dedication text here. Insert dedication text here. Insert dedication text here. Insert dedication text here. Insert dedication text here. Insert dedication text here.

A.I.D.S. Facts

A.I.D.S. Facts

.

A.I.D.S. Facts

ACKNOWLEDGMENTS

Insert acknowledgments text here. Insert acknowledgments text here. Insert acknowledgments text here. Insert acknowledgments text here. Insert acknowledgments text here. Insert acknowledgments text here. Insert acknowledgments text here. Insert acknowledgments text here. Insert acknowledgments text here. Insert acknowledgments text here.

A.I.D.S. Facts

A.I.D.S. Facts

Aids today

Neurological Complications of HIV

.

HIV is the virus that causes AIDS. HIV weakens and slowly destroys the body's immune system, leaving you vulnerable to life-threatening complications from an infection or the flu.

As HIV and AIDS battle your immune system, your central nervous system is also affected. HIV and AIDS both cause a number of neurological complications, particularly if HIV goes untreated and is allowed to progress to AIDS.

Today, antiretroviral medications—when taken correctly and promptly—help to slow down the progression of HIV and help ward off AIDS. Controlling HIV can also reduce your risk for neurological complications of HIV.

Facts about HIV/AIDS

HIV is a virus that's sexually transmitted, but can also be passed from mother to baby and person to person by sharing a contaminated needle or through transfusion of contaminated blood. Untreated, the virus will continue to replicate in the body, becoming more and more advanced. Advanced HIV becomes AIDS, which often results in a number of neurological complications as the body becomes more damaged.

HIV doesn't seem to take over the cells in your nervous system, but it does cause significant inflammation in the body. This inflammation can damage the spinal cord and brain and prevent your nerve cells from working the way that they should.

Neurological complications may result not only from damage caused by the virus itself, but also from other side effects of HIV and AIDS, such as cancers that are associated with these diseases. Some of the drugs used to treat HIV and AIDS can also cause neurological complications while attempting to control the rapid spread of the virus.

Neurological complications don't usually set in until HIV is advanced, typically when someone has AIDS. About half of adults with AIDS suffer from neurological complications related to HIV.

Types of neurological complications of HIV

HIV can cause many different conditions that affect the nervous system:

• Dementia. When HIV becomes very advanced, HIV-associated dementia or AIDS dementia complex can occur. These disorders impair cognitive function, which means that you may have trouble thinking, understanding, and remembering. This type of dementia can be life-threatening, but can often be prevented when antiretroviral drugs are taken correctly.

• Viral infections. HIV can increase your risk for several viral infections that strike the nervous system. Cytomegalovirus infections can negatively affect cognitive function, physical control (such as the use of legs and arms and bladder control), vision and hearing, and your respiratory system, causing problems like pneumonia. People with AIDS are also likely to develop a herpes virus infection such as shingles, inflammation in the brain, and inflammation in the spinal cord. Another condition, progressive multifocal leukoencephalopathy (PML) is also caused by a virus. PML is aggressive and dangerous but can be controlled with antiretroviral medications.

• Fungal and parasitic infections. Cryptococcal meningitis is caused by a fungus and leads to serious inflammation of the spinal cord and brain; it can be life-threatening if it isn't treated. A parasite can cause an infection called toxoplasma encephalitis, which often leads to confusion, seizures, and extremely painful headaches.

• Neuropathy. HIV can cause damage to nerves throughout the body, resulting in significant pain, known as neuropathy. Neuropathy is most common in people with advanced HIV.

• Vacuolar myelopathy. This condition occurs when tiny holes develop in the fibers of the nerves. It causes difficulty walking, particularly as the condition gets worse. It's common in people with AIDS who aren't receiving treatment and also in children with HIV.

• Psychological conditions. People with HIV or AIDS often develop anxiety disorders and suffer from depression. They may also experience hallucinations and significant changes in behavior.

• Lymphomas. Tumors called lymphomas often strike the brain of people with HIV. They're often related to another virus, similar to the herpes virus. Lymphomas can be life-threatening, but good management of HIV can make treating lymphomas more successful.

• Neurosyphilis. If an HIV-infected person also has syphilis that goes untreated, it can quickly progress and damage the nervous system. It can cause the nerve cells to break down and lead to loss of vision and hearing, dementia, and difficulty walking.

Symptoms

Once HIV begins affecting your immune system, it can cause many different symptoms. HIV-related neurological complications may lead to:

• Suddenly forgetting things all the time or acting confused

• Feeling of weakness that keeps getting worse

• Changes in behavior

• Headaches

- Problems with balance and coordination

- Seizures

- Changes in your vision

- Difficulty swallowing

- Losing feeling in your legs or arms

- Mental health problems like anxiety and depression

Diagnosis

Although a blood test can diagnose HIV and AIDS, a number of other diagnostic tests are needed to look at the different parts of the nervous system and diagnose neurological problems. Tests often include:

• An electromyography to measure the electrical activity of the muscles and nerves

• Biopsy to analyze a sample of tissues and help identify tumors in the brain or inflammation in the muscles

• Magnetic resonance spectroscopy. A test that examines the makeup of brain cells and that can help to tell the difference between abnormalities seen in the brain and spinal cord on MRI

• Sample of cerebrospinal fluid to look for infections, bleeding, or other abnormalities affecting the spinal cord or brain

• CT scan to look at the brain in great detail

• MRI, including standard and functional scans, to review damage to the brain and surrounding tissues

Treatment

Antiretroviral drugs are used to stop HIV from replicating and spreading throughout the body and to help reduce the risk that it will cause damage to the nervous system.

Specific neurological conditions and complications are treated differently. Cancer may be treated with chemotherapy and radiation, and bacterial infections need antibiotics. Certain medications may help manage viral infections, and medications to manage pain can help alleviate nerve pain. Counseling and medications, including antidepressants, may be used to manage some of the psychological conditions associated with HIV.

Prevention

Following all of your doctor's recommendations, especially taking all antiretroviral medications exactly as prescribed, can help control HIV and prevent its progression. Suppressing the virus with medications can help prevent damage to the body, including nervous system damage and neurological complications.

Managing HIV

Living a healthy lifestyle can help you better control HIV and prevent the progression to AIDS. Eating a healthy diet and maintaining a healthy body weight, exercising regularly, practicing safe sex, and following your medication regimen are all important steps in managing HIV.

Consult a doctor if you have a medical concern.

AIDS (acquired immune deficiency syndrome) is the final stage of HIV disease, which causes severe damage to the imm**Human immunodeficiency virus infection / acquired immunodeficiency syndrome (HIV/AIDS)** is a disease of the human immune system caused by infection with human immunodeficiency virus (HIV).[1] During the initial infection, a person may experience a brief period of influenza-like illness. This is typically followed by a prolonged period without symptoms. As the illness progresses, it interferes more and more with the immune system, making the person much more likely to get infections, including opportunistic infections and tumors that do not usually affect people who have working immune systems.

HIV is transmitted primarily via unprotected sexual intercourse (including anal and oral sex), contaminated blood transfusions, hypodermic needles, and from mother to child during pregnancy, delivery, or breastfeeding.[2] Some bodily fluids, such as saliva and tears, do not transmit HIV.[3] Prevention of HIV infection, primarily through safe sex and needle-exchange programs, is a key strategy to control the spread of the disease. There is no cure or vaccine; however, antiretroviral treatment can slow the course of the disease and may lead to a near-normal life expectancy. While antiretroviral treatment reduces the risk of death and complications from the disease, these medications are expensive and have side effects. Without treatment, the average survival time after infection with HIV is estimated to be 9 to 11 years, depending on the HIV subtype.[4]

Genetic research indicates that HIV originated in west-central Africa during the late nineteenth or early twentieth century.[5] AIDS was first recognized by the United States Centers for Disease Control and Prevention (CDC) in 1981 and its cause— HIV infection—was identified in the early part of the decade.[6] Since its discovery, AIDS has caused an estimated 36 million deaths worldwide (as of 2012).[7] As of 2012, approximately 35.3 million people are living with HIV globally.[7] HIV/AIDS is considered a pandemic—a disease outbreak which is present over a large area and is actively spreading.[8]

HIV/AIDS has had a great impact on society, both as an illness and as a source of discrimination. The disease also has significant economic impacts. There are many misconceptions about HIV/AIDS such as the belief that it can be transmitted by casual non-sexual contact. The disease has also become subject to many controversies involving religion. It has attracted international medical and political attention as well as large-scale funding since it was identified in the 1980s.[9]

Contents

[hide]

Signs and symptoms

Main article: Signs and symptoms of HIV/AIDS

There are three main stages of HIV infection: acute infection, clinical latency and AIDS.[10][11]

Acute infection

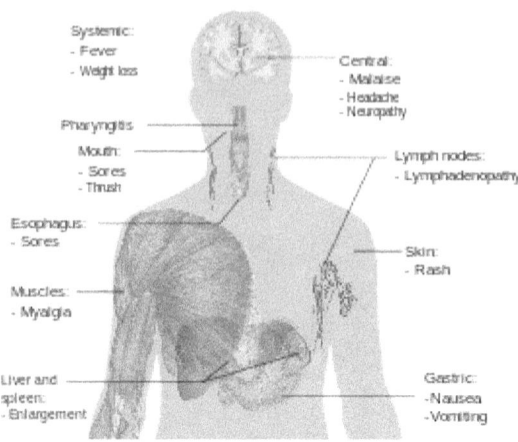

Main symptoms of acute HIV infection

The initial period following the contraction of HIV is called acute HIV, primary HIV or acute retroviral syndrome.[10][12] Many individuals develop an influenza-like illness or a mononucleosis-like illness 2–4 weeks post exposure while others have no significant symptoms.[13][14] Symptoms occur in 40–90% of cases and most commonly include fever, large tender lymph nodes, throat inflammation, a rash, headache, and/or sores of the mouth and genitals.[12][14] The rash, which occurs in 20–50% of cases, presents itself on the trunk and is maculopapular, classically.[15] Some people also develop opportunistic infections at this stage.[12] Gastrointestinal symptoms such as nausea, vomiting or diarrhea may occur, as may neurological symptoms of peripheral neuropathy or Guillain-Barre syndrome.[14] The duration of the symptoms varies, but is usually one or two weeks.[14]

Due to their nonspecific character, these symptoms are not often recognized as signs of HIV infection. Even cases that do get seen by a family doctor or a hospital are often misdiagnosed as one of the many common infectious diseases with overlapping symptoms. Thus, it is recommended that HIV be considered in people presenting an unexplained fever who may have risk factors for the infection.[14]

Clinical latency

The initial symptoms are followed by a stage called clinical latency, asymptomatic HIV, or chronic HIV.[11] Without treatment, this second stage of the natural history of HIV infection can last from about three years[16] to over 20 years[17] (on average, about eight years).[18] While typically there are few or no symptoms at first, near the end of this stage many people experience fever, weight loss, gastrointestinal problems and muscle pains.[11] Between 50 and 70% of people also develop persistent generalized lymphadenopathy, characterized by unexplained, non-painful enlargement of more than one group of lymph nodes (other than in the groin) for over three to six months.[10]

Although most HIV-1 infected individuals have a detectable viral load and in the absence of treatment will eventually progress to AIDS, a small proportion (about 5%) retain high levels of CD4$^+$ T cells (T helper cells) without antiretroviral therapy for more than 5 years.[14][19] These individuals are classified as HIV controllers or long-term nonprogressors (LTNP).[19] Another group is those who also maintain a low or undctcctable viral load without anti-retroviral treatment who are known as "elite controllers" or "elite suppressors". They represent approximately 1 in 300 infected persons.[20]

Acquired immunodeficiency syndrome

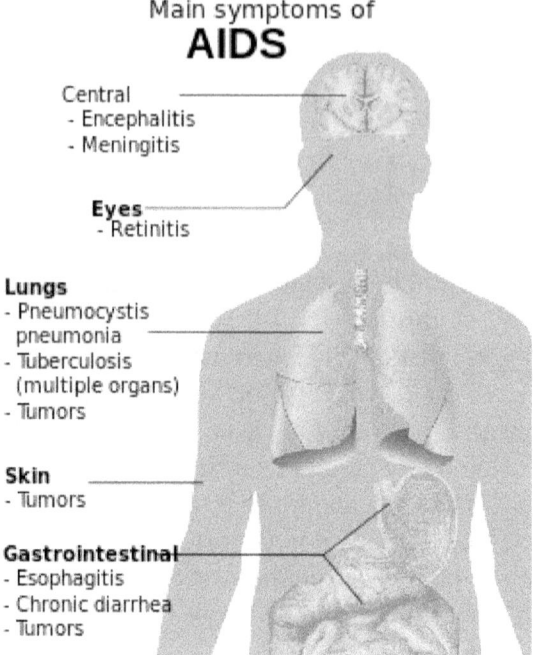

Main symptoms of AIDS.

Acquired immunodeficiency syndrome (AIDS) is defined in terms of either a CD4$^+$ T cell count below 200 cells per μL or the occurrence of specific diseases in association with an HIV infection.[14] In the absence of specific treatment, around half of people infected with HIV develop AIDS within ten years.[14] The most common initial conditions that alert to the presence of AIDS are pneumocystis pneumonia (40%), cachexia in the form of HIV wasting syndrome (20%) and esophageal candidiasis.[14] Other common signs include recurring respiratory tract infections.[14]

Opportunistic infections may be caused by bacteria, viruses, fungi and parasites that are normally controlled by the immune system.[21] Which infections occur partly depends on what organisms are common in the person's environment.[14] These infections may affect nearly every organ system.[22]

People with AIDS have an increased risk of developing various viral induced cancers including Kaposi's sarcoma, Burkitt's lymphoma, primary central nervous system lymphoma, and cervical cancer.[15] Kaposi's sarcoma is the most common cancer occurring in 10 to 20% of people with HIV.[23] The second most common cancer is lymphoma which is the cause of death of nearly 16% of people with AIDS and is the initial sign of AIDS in 3 to 4%.[23] Both these cancers are associated with human herpesvirus 8.[23] Cervical cancer occurs more frequently in those with AIDS due to its association with human papillomavirus (HPV).[23]

Additionally, people with AIDS frequently have systemic symptoms such as prolonged fevers, sweats (particularly at night), swollen lymph nodes, chills, weakness, and weight loss.[24] Diarrhea is another common symptom present in about 90% of people with AIDS.[25] They can also be affected by diverse psychiatric and neurological symptoms independent of opportunistic infections and cancers.[26]

Transmission

Average per act risk of getting HIV by exposure route to an infected source	
Exposure route	**Chance of infection**
Blood transfusion	90% [27]
Childbirth (to child)	25%[28]
Needle-sharing injection drug use	0.67%[27]
Percutaneous needle stick	0.30%[29]
Receptive anal intercourse*	0.04–3.0%[30]
Insertive anal intercourse*	0.03%[31]
Receptive penile-vaginal intercourse*	0.05–0.30%[30][32]
Insertive penile-vaginal intercourse*	0.01–0.38% [30][32]
Receptive oral intercourse*§	0–0.04% [30]
Insertive oral intercourse*§	0–0.005%[33]

* assuming no condom use
§ source refers to oral intercourse performed on a man

HIV is transmitted by three main routes: sexual contact, exposure to infected body fluids or tissues, and from mother to child during pregnancy, delivery, or breastfeeding (known as vertical transmission).[2] There is no risk of acquiring HIV if exposed to feces, nasal secretions, saliva, sputum, sweat, tears, urine, or vomit unless these are contaminated with blood.[29] It is possible to be co-infected by more than one strain of HIV—a condition known as HIV superinfection.[34]

Sexual

The most frequent mode of transmission of HIV is through sexual contact with an infected person.[2] The majority of all transmissions worldwide occur through heterosexual contacts (i.e. sexual contacts between people of the opposite sex);[2] however, the pattern of transmission varies significantly among countries. In the United States, as of 2009, most sexual transmission occurred in men who had sex with men,[2] with this population accounting for 64% of all new cases.[35]

As regards unprotected heterosexual contacts, estimates of the risk of HIV transmission per sexual act appear to be four to ten times higher in low-income countries than in high-income countries.[36] In low-income countries, the risk of female-to-male transmission is estimated as 0.38% per act, and of male-to-female transmission as 0.30% per act; the equivalent estimates for high-income countries are 0.04% per act for female-to-male transmission, and 0.08% per act for male-to-female transmission.[36] The risk of transmission from anal intercourse is especially high, estimated as 1.4–1.7% per act in both heterosexual and homosexual contacts.[36][37] While the risk of transmission from oral sex is relatively low, it is still present.[38] The risk from receiving oral sex has been described as "nearly nil"[39] however a few cases have been reported.[40] The per-act risk is estimated at 0–0.04% for receptive oral intercourse.[41] In settings involving prostitution in low income countries, risk of female-to-male transmission has been estimated as 2.4% per act and male-to-female transmission as 0.05% per act.[36]

Risk of transmission increases in the presence of many sexually transmitted infections[42] and genital ulcers.[36] Genital ulcers appear to increase the risk approximately fivefold.[36] Other sexually transmitted infections, such as gonorrhea, chlamydia, trichomoniasis, and bacterial vaginosis, are associated with somewhat smaller increases in risk of transmission.[41]

The viral load of an infected person is an important risk factor in both sexual and mother-to-child transmission.[43] During the first 2.5 months of an HIV infection a person's infectiousness is twelve times higher due to this high viral load.[41] If the person is in the late stages of infection, rates of transmission are approximately eightfold greater.[36]

Commercial sex workers (including those in pornography) have an increased rate of HIV.[44][45] Rough sex can be a factor associated with an increased risk of transmission.[46] Sexual assault is also believed to carry an increased risk of HIV transmission as condoms are rarely worn, physical trauma to the vagina or rectum is likely, and there may be a greater risk of concurrent sexually transmitted infections.[47]

Body fluids

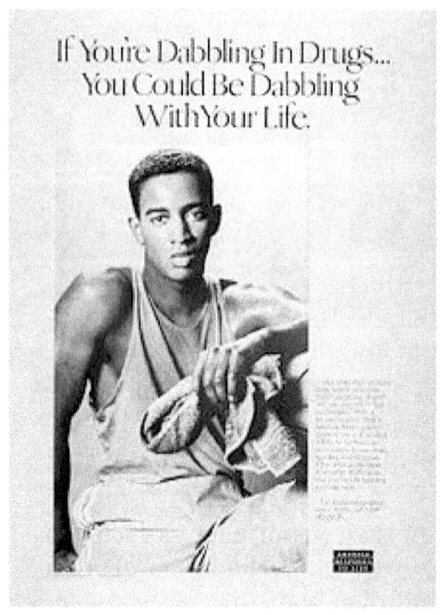

CDC poster from 1989 highlighting the threat of AIDS associated with drug use

The second most frequent mode of HIV transmission is via blood and blood products.[2] Blood-borne transmission can be through needle-sharing during intravenous drug use, needle stick injury, transfusion of contaminated blood or blood product, or medical injections with unsterilised equipment. The risk from sharing a needle during drug injection is between 0.63 and 2.4% per act, with an average of 0.8%.[48] The risk of acquiring HIV from a needle stick from an HIV-infected person is estimated as 0.3% (about 1 in 333) per act and the risk following mucous membrane exposure to infected blood as 0.09% (about 1 in 1000) per act.[29] In the United States intravenous drug users made up 12% of all new cases of HIV in 2009,[35] and in some areas more than 80% of people who inject drugs are HIV positive.[2]

HIV is transmitted in about 93% of blood transfusions involving infected blood.[48] In developed countries the risk of acquiring HIV from a blood transfusion is extremely low (less than one in half a million) where improved donor selection and HIV screening is performed;[2] for example, in the UK the risk is reported at one in five million.[49] In low income countries, only half of transfusions may be appropriately screened (as of 2008),[50] and it is estimated that up to 15% of HIV infections in these areas come from transfusion of infected blood and blood products, representing between 5% and 10% of global infections.[2][51]

Unsafe medical injections play a significant role in HIV spread in sub-Saharan Africa. In 2007, between 12 and 17% of infections in this region were attributed to medical syringe use.[52] The World Health Organisation estimates the risk of transmission as a result of a medical injection in Africa at 1.2%.[52] Significant risks are also associated with invasive procedures, assisted delivery, and dental care in this area of the world.[52]

People giving or receiving tattoos, piercings, and scarification are theoretically at risk of infection but no confirmed cases have been documented.[53] It is not possible for mosquitoes or other insects to transmit HIV.[54]

Mother-to-child

HIV can be transmitted from mother to child during pregnancy, during delivery, or through breast milk.[55][56] This is the third most common way in which HIV is transmitted globally.[2] In the absence of treatment, the risk of transmission before or during birth is around 20% and in those who also breastfeed 35%.[55] As of 2008, vertical transmission accounted for about 90% of cases of HIV in children.[55] With appropriate treatment the risk of mother-to-child infection can be reduced to about 1%.[55] Preventive treatment involves the mother taking antiretroviral during pregnancy and delivery, an elective caesarean section, avoiding breastfeeding, and administering antiretroviral drugs to the newborn.[57] Many of these measures are however not available in the developing world.[57] If blood contaminates food during pre-chewing it may pose a risk of transmission.[53]

Virology

Main article: HIV

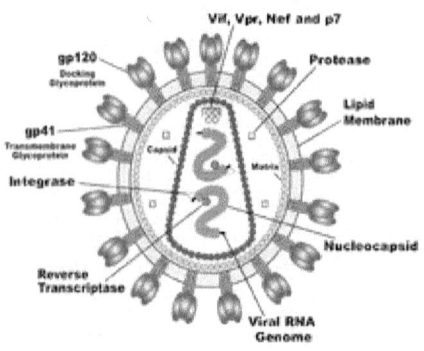

A diagram showing the structure of HIV virus

HIV is the cause of the spectrum of disease known as HIV/AIDS. HIV is a retrovirus that primarily infects components of the human immune system such as CD4⁺ T cells, macrophages and dendritic cells. It directly and indirectly destroys CD4⁺ T cells.[58]

HIV is a member of the genus *Lentivirus*,[59] part of the family *Retroviridae*.[60] Lentiviruses share many morphological and biological characteristics. Many species of mammals are infected by lentiviruses, which are characteristically responsible for long-duration illnesses with a long incubation period.[61] Lentiviruses are transmitted as single-stranded, positive-sense, enveloped RNA viruses. Upon entry into the target cell, the viral RNA genome is converted (reverse transcribed) into double-stranded DNA by a virally encoded reverse transcriptase that is transported along with the viral genome in the virus particle. The resulting viral DNA is then imported into the cell nucleus and integrated into the cellular DNA by a virally encoded integrase and host co-factors.[62] Once integrated, the virus may become latent, allowing the virus and its host cell to avoid detection by the immune system.[63] Alternatively, the virus may be transcribed, producing new RNA genomes and viral proteins that are packaged and released from the cell as new virus particles that begin the replication cycle anew.[64]

Two types of HIV have been characterized: HIV-1 and HIV-2. HIV-1 is the virus that was originally discovered (and initially referred to also as LAV or HTLV-III). It is more <u>virulent</u>, more <u>infective</u>,[65] and is the cause of the majority of HIV infections globally. The lower infectivity of HIV-2 as compared with HIV-1 implies that fewer people exposed to HIV-2 will be infected per exposure. Because of its relatively poor capacity for transmission, HIV-2 is largely confined to <u>West Africa</u>.[66]

Pathophysiology

Main article: <u>Pathophysiology of HIV/AIDS</u>

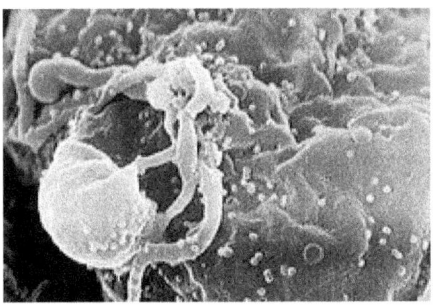

<u>Scanning electron micrograph</u> of HIV-1, colored green, budding from a cultured <u>lymphocyte</u>.

After the virus enters the body there is a period of rapid <u>viral replication</u>, leading to an abundance of virus in the peripheral blood. During primary infection, the level of HIV may reach several million virus particles per milliliter of blood.[67] This response is accompanied by a marked drop in the number of circulating CD4+ T cells. The acute <u>viremia</u> is almost invariably associated with activation of <u>CD8+ T cells</u>, which kill HIV-infected cells, and subsequently with antibody production, or <u>seroconversion</u>. The CD8+ T cell response is thought to be important in controlling virus levels, which peak and then decline, as the CD4+ T cell counts recover. A good CD8+ T cell response has been linked to slower disease progression and a better prognosis, though it does not eliminate the virus.[68]

Ultimately, HIV causes AIDS by depleting <u>CD4+ T cells</u>. This weakens the immune system and allows <u>opportunistic infections</u>. T cells are essential to the immune response and without them, the body cannot fight infections or kill cancerous cells. The mechanism of CD4+ T cell depletion differs in the acute and chronic phases.[69] During the acute phase, HIV-induced cell lysis and killing of infected cells by cytotoxic T cells accounts for CD4+ T cell depletion, although apoptosis may also be a factor. During the chronic phase, the consequences of generalized immune activation coupled with the gradual loss of the ability of the immune system to generate new T cells appear to account for the slow decline in CD4+ T cell numbers.[70]

Although the symptoms of immune deficiency characteristic of AIDS do not appear for years after a person is infected, the bulk of CD4+ T cell loss occurs during the first weeks of infection, especially in the intestinal mucosa, which harbors the majority of the lymphocytes found in the body.[71] The reason for the preferential loss of mucosal CD4+ T cells is that the majority of mucosal CD4+ T cells express the CCR5 protein which HIV uses as a co-receptor to gain access to the cells, whereas only a small fraction of CD4+ T cells in the bloodstream do so.[72] A specific genetic change that alters the CCR5 protein when present in both chromosomes very effectively prevents HIV-1 infection.[73]

HIV seeks out and destroys CCR5 expressing CD4+ T cells during acute infection.[74] A vigorous immune response eventually controls the infection and initiates the clinically latent phase. CD4+ T cells in mucosal tissues remain particularly affected.[74] Continuous HIV replication causes a state of generalized immune activation persisting throughout the chronic phase.[75] Immune activation, which is reflected by the increased activation state of immune cells and release of pro-inflammatory cytokines, results from the activity of several HIV gene products and the immune response to ongoing HIV replication. It is also linked to the breakdown of the immune surveillance system of the gastrointestinal mucosal barrier caused by the depletion of mucosal CD4+ T cells during the acute phase of disease.[76]

Diagnosis

Main article: <u>*Diagnosis of HIV/AIDS*</u>

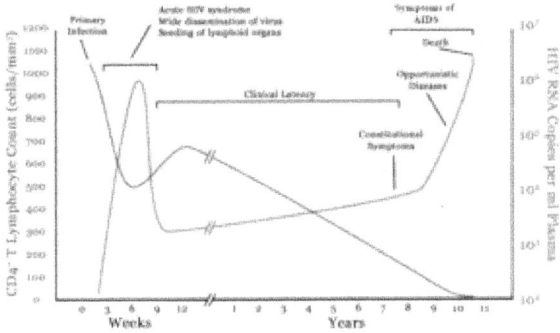

A generalized graph of the relationship between HIV copies (viral load) and CD4⁺ T cell counts over the average course of untreated HIV infection. ⬜ CD4⁺ T Lymphocyte count (cells/mm³) ⬜ HIV RNA copies per mL of plasma

HIV/AIDS is diagnosed via laboratory testing and then staged based on the presence of <u>certain signs or symptoms</u>.[12] HIV screening is recommended by the <u>United States Preventive Services Task Force</u> for all people 15 years to 65 years of age including all pregnant women.[77] Additionally testing is recommended for all those at high risk, which includes anyone diagnosed with a sexually transmitted illness.[15] In many areas of the world a third of HIV carriers only discover they are infected at an advanced stage of the disease when AIDS or severe immunodeficiency has become apparent.[15]

HIV testing

Most people infected with HIV develop specific <u>antibodies</u> (i.e. <u>seroconvert</u>) within three to twelve weeks of the initial infection.[14] Diagnosis of primary HIV before seroconversion is done by measuring HIV-<u>RNA</u> or <u>p24 antigen</u>.[14] Positive results obtained by antibody or <u>PCR</u> testing are confirmed either by a different antibody or by PCR.[12]

Antibody tests in children younger than 18 months are typically inaccurate due to the continued presence of <u>maternal antibodies</u>.[78]

Thus HIV infection can only be diagnosed by PCR testing for HIV RNA or DNA, or via testing for the p24 antigen.[12] Much of the world lacks access to reliable PCR testing and many places simply wait until either symptoms develop or the child is old enough for accurate antibody testing.[78] In sub-Saharan Africa as of 2007–2009 between 30 and 70% of the population was aware of their HIV status.[79] In 2009, between 3.6 and 42% of men and women in Sub-Saharan countries were tested[79] which represented a significant increase compared to previous years.[79]

Classifications of HIV infection

Two main clinical staging systems are used to classify HIV and HIV-related disease for surveillance purposes: the WHO disease staging system for HIV infection and disease,[12] and the CDC classification system for HIV infection.[80] The CDC's classification system is more frequently adopted in developed countries. Since the WHO's staging system does not require laboratory tests, it is suited to the resource-restricted conditions encountered in developing countries, where it can also be used to help guide clinical management. Despite their differences, the two systems allow comparison for statistical purposes.[10][12][80]

The World Health Organization first proposed a definition for AIDS in 1986.[12] Since then, the WHO classification has been updated and expanded several times, with the most recent version being published in 2007.[12] The WHO system uses the following categories:

- Primary HIV infection: May be either asymptomatic or associated with acute retroviral syndrome.[12]
- Stage I: HIV infection is asymptomatic with a CD4$^+$ T cell count (also known as CD4 count) greater than 500 per microlitre (μl or cubic mm) of blood.[12] May include generalized lymph node enlargement.[12]
- Stage II: Mild symptoms which may include minor mucocutaneous manifestations and recurrent upper

respiratory tract infections. A CD4 count of less than 500/μl.[12]

- Stage III: Advanced symptoms which may include unexplained chronic diarrhea for longer than a month, severe bacterial infections including tuberculosis of the lung, and a CD4 count of less than 350/μl.[12]
- Stage IV or AIDS: severe symptoms which include toxoplasmosis of the brain, candidiasis of the esophagus, trachea, bronchi or lungs and Kaposi's sarcoma. A CD4 count of less than 200/μl.[12]

The United States Center for Disease Control and Prevention also created a classification system for HIV, and updated it in 2008.[80] This system classifies HIV infections based on CD4 count and clinical symptoms,[80] and describes the infection in three stages:

- Stage 1: CD4 count ≥ 500 cells/μl and no AIDS defining conditions
- Stage 2: CD4 count 200 to 500 cells/μl and no AIDS defining conditions
- Stage 3: CD4 count ≤ 200 cells/μl or AIDS defining conditions
- Unknown: if insufficient information is available to make any of the above classifications

For surveillance purposes, the AIDS diagnosis still stands even if, after treatment, the CD4+ T cell count rises to above 200 per μL of blood or other AIDS-defining illnesses are cured.[10]

Prevention

Main article: Prevention of HIV/AIDS

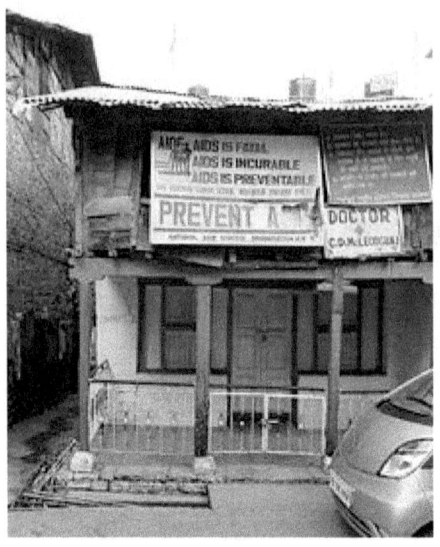

AIDS Clinic, McLeod Ganj, Himachal Pradesh, India, 2010

Sexual contact

Consistent condom use reduces the risk of HIV transmission by approximately 80% over the long term.[81] When condoms are used consistently by a couple in which one person is infected, the rate of HIV infection is less than 1% per year.[82] There is some evidence to suggest that female condoms may provide an equivalent level of protection.[83] Application of a vaginal gel containing tenofovir (a reverse transcriptase inhibitor) immediately before sex seems to reduce infection rates by approximately 40% among African women.[84] By contrast, use of the spermicide nonoxynol-9 may increase the risk of transmission due to its tendency to cause vaginal and rectal irritation.[85] Circumcision in Sub-Saharan Africa "reduces the acquisition of HIV by heterosexual men by between 38% and 66% over 24 months".[86] Based on these studies, the World Health Organization and UNAIDS both recommended male circumcision as a method of preventing female-to-male HIV transmission in 2007.[87] Whether it protects against male-to-female transmission is disputed[88][89] and whether it is of benefit in developed countries and among men who have sex with men is undetermined.[90][91][92] Some experts fear that a lower perception of vulnerability among circumcised men may cause more sexual risk-taking behavior, thus negating its preventive effects.[93]

Programs encouraging sexual abstinence do not appear to affect subsequent HIV risk.[94] Evidence for a benefit from peer education is equally poor.[95] Comprehensive sexual education provided at school may decrease high risk behavior.[96] A substantial minority of young people continues to engage in high-risk practices despite knowing about HIV/AIDS, underestimating their own risk of becoming infected with HIV.[97] It is not known whether treating other sexually transmitted infections is effective in preventing HIV.[42]

Pre-exposure

Treating people with HIV whose CD4 count ≥ 350cells/μL with antiretrovirals protects 96% of their partners from infection.[98] This is about a 10 to 20 fold reduction in transmission risk.[99] Pre-exposure prophylaxis (PrEP) with a daily dose of the medications tenofovir, with or without emtricitabine, is effective in a number of groups including men who have sex with men, couples where one is HIV positive, and young heterosexuals in Africa.[84] It may also be effective in intravenous drug users with a study finding a decrease in risk of 0.7 to 0.4 per 100 person years.[100]

Universal precautions within the health care environment are believed to be effective in decreasing the risk of HIV.[101] Intravenous drug use is an important risk factor and harm reduction strategies such as needle-exchange programmes and opioid substitution therapy appear effective in decreasing this risk.[102][103]

Post-exposure

A course of antiretrovirals administered within 48 to 72 hours after exposure to HIV-positive blood or genital secretions is referred to as post-exposure prophylaxis (PEP).[104] The use of the single agent zidovudine reduces the risk of a HIV infection five-fold following a needle-stick injury.[104] As of 2013, the prevention regimen recommended in the United States consists of three medications—tenofovir, emtricitabine and raltegravir—as this may reduce the risk further.[105]

PEP treatment is recommended after a sexual assault when the perpetrator is known to be HIV positive, but is controversial when their HIV status is unknown.[106] The duration of treatment is usually four weeks[107] and is frequently associated with adverse effects—where zidovudine is used, about 70% of cases result in adverse effects such as nausea (24%), fatigue (22%), emotional distress (13%) and headaches (9%).[29]

Mother-to-child

Programs to prevent the vertical transmission of HIV (from mothers to children) can reduce rates of transmission by 92–99%.[55][102] This primarily involves the use of a combination of antiviral medications during pregnancy and after birth in the infant and potentially includes bottle feeding rather than breastfeeding.[55][108] If replacement feeding is acceptable, feasible, affordable, sustainable, and safe, mothers should avoid breastfeeding their infants; however exclusive breastfeeding is recommended during the first months of life if this is not the case.[109] If exclusive breastfeeding is carried out, the provision of extended antiretroviral prophylaxis to the infant decreases the risk of transmission.[110]

Vaccination

Main article: HIV vaccine

As of 2012 there is no effective vaccine for HIV or AIDS.[111] A single trial of the vaccine RV 144 published in 2009 found a partial reduction in the risk of transmission of roughly 30%, stimulating some hope in the research community of developing a truly effective vaccine.[112] Further trials of the RV 144 vaccine are ongoing.[113][114]

Management

Main article: Management of HIV/AIDS

There is currently no cure or effective HIV vaccine. Treatment consists of high active antiretroviral therapy (HAART) which slows progression of the disease[115] and as of 2010 more than 6.6 million people were taking them in low and middle income countries.[116] Treatment also includes preventive and active treatment of opportunistic infections.

Antiviral therapy

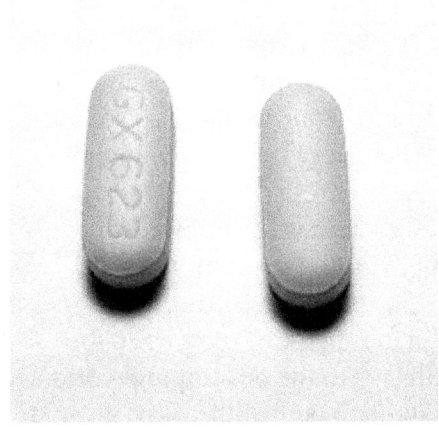

Abacavir – a nucleoside analog reverse transcriptase inhibitor (NARTI or NRTI)

Current HAART options are combinations (or "cocktails") consisting of at least three medications belonging to at least two types, or "classes," of antiretroviral agents.[117] Initially treatment is typically a non-nucleoside reverse transcriptase inhibitor (NNRTI) plus two nucleoside analogue reverse transcriptase inhibitors (NRTIs).[118] Typical NRTIs include: zidovudine (AZT) or tenofovir (TDF) and lamivudine (3TC) or emtricitabine (FTC).[118] Combinations of agents which include a protease inhibitors (PI) are used if the above regimen loses effectiveness.[117]

When to start antiretroviral therapy is subject to debate.[15][119] The World Health Organization recommends antiretrovirals in all adolescents, adults and pregnant women with a CD4 count less than 500/µl with this being especially important in those with counts less than 350/µl or those with symptoms regardless of CD4 count.[118] This is supported by the fact that beginning treatment at this level reduces the risk of death.[120] The United States in addition recommends them for all HIV-infected people regardless of CD4 count or symptoms; however it makes this recommendation with less confidence for those with higher counts.[121] While the WHO also recommends treatment in those who are co-infected with tuberculosis and those with chronic active hepatitis B.[117] Once treatment is begun it is recommended that it is continued without breaks or "holidays".[15] Many people are diagnosed only after treatment ideally should have begun.[15] The desired outcome of treatment is a long term plasma HIV-RNA count below 50 copies/mL.[15] Levels to determine if treatment is effective are initially recommended after four weeks and once levels fall below 50 copies/mL checks every three to six months are typically adequate.[15] Inadequate control is deemed to be greater than 400 copies/mL.[15] Based on these criteria treatment is effective in more than 95% of people during the first year.[15]

Benefits of treatment include a decreased risk of progression to AIDS and a decreased risk of death.[122] In the developing world treatment also improves physical and mental health.[123] With treatment there is a 70% reduced risk of acquiring tuberculosis.[117] Additional benefits include a decreased risk of transmission of the disease to sexual partners and a decrease in mother-to-child transmission.[117] The effectiveness of treatment depends to a large part on compliance.[15] Reasons for non-adherence include poor access to medical care,[124] inadequate social supports, mental illness and drug abuse.[125] The complexity of treatment regimens (due to pill numbers and dosing frequency) and adverse effects may reduce adherence.[126] Even though cost is an important issue with some medications,[127] 47% of those who needed them were taking them in low and middle income countries as of 2010[116] and the rate of adherence is similar in low-income and high-income countries.[128]

Specific adverse events are related to the antiretroviral agent taken.[129] Some relatively common adverse events include: lipodystrophy syndrome, dyslipidemia, and diabetes mellitus, especially with protease inhibitors.[10] Other common symptoms include diarrhea,[129][130] and an increased risk of cardiovascular disease.[131] Newer recommended treatments are associated with fewer adverse effects.[15] Certain medications may be associated with birth defects and therefore may be unsuitable for women hoping to have children.[15]

Treatment recommendations for children are slightly different from those for adults. In the developing world, as of 2010, 23% of children who were in need of treatment had access.[132] Both the World Health Organization and the United States recommend treatment for all children less than twelve months of age.[133][134] The United States recommends in those between one year and five years of age treatment in those with HIV RNA counts of greater than 100,000 copies/mL, and in those more than five years treatments when CD4 counts are less than 500/µl.[133]

Opportunistic infections

Measures to prevent opportunistic infections are effective in many people with HIV/AIDS. In addition to improving current disease, treatment with antiretrovirals reduces the risk of developing additional opportunistic infections.[129] Vaccination against hepatitis A and B is advised for all people at risk of HIV before they become infected; however it may also be given after infection.[135] Trimethoprim/sulfamethoxazole prophylaxis between four and six weeks of age and ceasing breastfeeding in infants born to HIV positive mothers is recommended in resource limited settings.[132] It is also recommended to prevent PCP when a person's CD4 count is below 200 cells/uL and in those who have or have previously had PCP.[136] People with substantial immunosuppression are also advised to receive prophylactic therapy for toxoplasmosis and Cryptococcus meningitis.[137] Appropriate preventive measures have reduced the rate of these infections by 50% between 1992 and 1997.[138]

Alternative medicine

In the US, approximately 60% of people with HIV use various forms of complementary or alternative medicine,[139] even though the effectiveness of most of these therapies has not been established.[140] With respect to dietary advice and AIDS some evidence has shown a benefit from micronutrient supplements.[141] Evidence for supplementation with selenium is mixed with some tentative evidence of benefit.[142] There is some evidence that vitamin A supplementation in children reduces mortality and improves growth.[141] In Africa in nutritionally compromised pregnant and lactating women a multivitamin supplementation has improved outcomes for both mothers and children.[141] Dietary intake of micronutrients at RDA levels by HIV-infected adults is recommended by the World Health Organization.[143][144] The WHO further states that several studies indicate that supplementation of vitamin A, zinc, and iron can produce adverse effects in HIV positive adults.[144] There is not enough evidence to support the use of herbal medicines.[145]

Prognosis

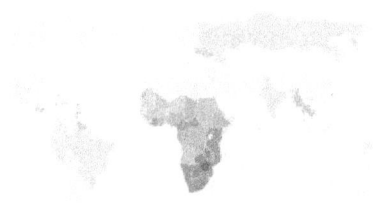

Disability-adjusted life year for HIV and AIDS per 100,000 inhabitants as of 2004.

no data	1000–2500
≤ 10	2500–5000
10–25	5000–7500
25–50	7500-10000
50–100	10000-50000
100–500	≥ 50000
500–1000	

HIV/AIDS has become a chronic rather than an acutely fatal disease in many areas of the world.[146] Prognosis varies between people, and both the CD4 count and viral load are useful for predicted outcomes.[14] Without treatment, average survival time after infection with HIV is estimated to be 9 to 11 years, depending on the HIV subtype.[4] After the diagnosis of AIDS, if treatment is not available, survival ranges between 6 and 19 months.[147][148] HAART and appropriate prevention of opportunistic infections reduces the death rate by 80%, and raises the life expectancy for a newly diagnosed young adult to 20–50 years.[146][149][150] This is between two thirds[149] and nearly that of the general population.[15][151] If treatment is started late in the infection, prognosis is not as good:[15] for example, if treatment is begun following the diagnosis of AIDS, life expectancy is ~10–40 years.[15][146] Half of infants born with HIV die before two years of age without treatment.[132]

The primary causes of death from HIV/AIDS are opportunistic infections and cancer, both of which are frequently the result of the progressive failure of the immune system.[138][152] Risk of cancer appears to increase once the CD4 count is below 500/μL.[15] The rate of clinical disease progression varies widely between individuals and has been shown to be affected by a number of factors such as a person's susceptibility and immune function;[153] their access to health care, the presence of co-infections;[147][154] and the particular strain (or strains) of the virus involved.[155][156]

Tuberculosis co-infection is one of the leading causes of sickness and death in those with HIV/AIDS being present in a third of all HIV infected people and causing 25% of HIV related deaths.[157] HIV is also one of the most important risk factors for tuberculosis.[158] Hepatitis C is another very common co-infection where each disease increases the progression of the other.[159] The two most common cancers associated with HIV/AIDS are Kaposi's sarcoma and AIDS-related non-Hodgkin's lymphoma.[152]

Even with anti-retroviral treatment, over the long term HIV-infected people may experience neurocognitive disorders,[160] osteoporosis,[161] neuropathy,[162] cancers,[163][164] nephropathy,[165] and cardiovascular disease.[130] It is not clear whether these conditions result from the HIV infection itself or are adverse effects of treatment.

Epidemiology

Main article: Epidemiology of HIV/AIDS

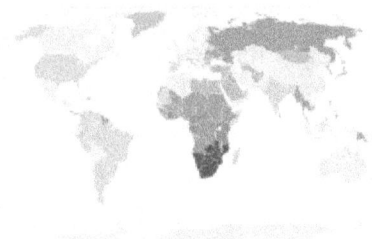

Estimated prevalence in % of HIV among young adults (15–49) per country as of 2011.[166]

No data	1–5
<0.10	5–15
0.10–0.5	15–50
0.5–1	

HIV/AIDS is a global pandemic.[167] As of 2012, approximately 35.3 million people have HIV worldwide with the number of new infections that year being about 2.3 million.[168] This is down from 3.1 million new infections in 2001.[168] Of these approximately 16.8 million are women and 3.4 million are less than 15 years old.[116] It resulted in about 1.6 million deaths in 2012, down from a peak of 2.2 million in 2005.[116][168]

Sub-Saharan Africa is the region most affected. In 2010, an estimated 68% (22.9 million) of all HIV cases and 66% of all deaths (1.2 million) occurred in this region.[169] This means that about 5% of the adult population is infected[170] and it is believed to be the cause of 10% of all deaths in children.[171] Here in contrast to other regions women compose nearly 60% of cases.[169]

South Africa has the largest population of people with HIV of any country in the world at 5.9 million.[169] Life expectancy has fallen in the worst-affected countries due to HIV/AIDS; for example, in 2006 it was estimated that it had dropped from 65 to 35 years in Botswana.[8] Mother-to-child transmission, as of 2013, in Botswana and South Africa has decreased to less than 5% with improvement in many other African nations due to improved access to antiretroviral therapy.[172]

South & South East Asia is the second most affected; in 2010 this region contained an estimated 4 million cases or 12% of all people living with HIV resulting in approximately 250,000 deaths.[170] Approximately 2.4 million of these cases are in India.[169]

In 2008 in the United States approximately 1.2 million people were living with HIV, resulting in about 17,500 deaths. The US Centers for Disease Control and Prevention estimated that in 2008 20% of infected Americans were unaware of their infection.[173] In the United Kingdom as of 2009 there were approximately 86,500 cases which resulted in 516 deaths.[174] In Canada as of 2008 there were about 65,000 cases causing 53 deaths.[175] Between the first recognition of AIDS in 1981 and 2009 it has led to nearly 30 million deaths.[176] Prevalence is lowest in Middle East and North Africa at 0.1% or less, East Asia at 0.1% and Western and Central Europe at 0.2%.[170] The worst affected European countries in 2009 are Estonia, Ukraine, Russia, Latvia and Portugal.[177]

History

Main article: History of HIV/AIDS

Discovery

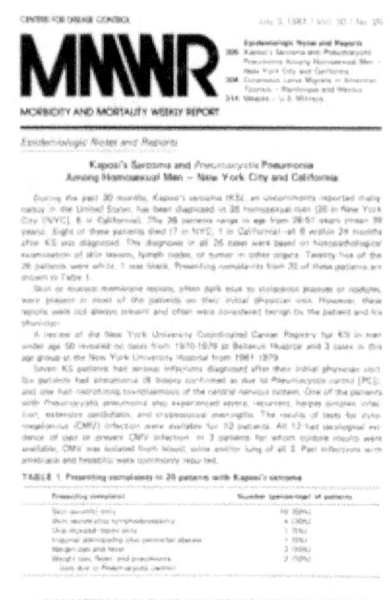

The *Morbidity and Mortality Weekly Report* reported in 1981 on what was later to be called "AIDS".

AIDS was first clinically observed in 1981 in the United States.[23] The initial cases were a cluster of injecting drug users and homosexual men with no known cause of impaired immunity who showed symptoms of *Pneumocystis carinii* pneumonia (PCP), a rare opportunistic infection that was known to occur in people with very compromised immune systems.[178] Soon thereafter, an unexpected number of gay men developed a previously rare skin cancer called Kaposi's sarcoma (KS).[179][180] Many more cases of PCP and KS emerged, alerting U.S. Centers for Disease Control and Prevention (CDC) and a CDC task force was formed to monitor the outbreak.[181]

In the early days, the CDC did not have an official name for the disease, often referring to it by way of the diseases that were associated with it, for example, lymphadenopathy, the disease after which the discoverers of HIV originally named the virus.[182][183] They also used *Kaposi's Sarcoma and Opportunistic Infections*, the name by which a task force had been set up in 1981.[184] At one point, the CDC coined the phrase "the 4H disease", since the syndrome seemed to affect <u>Haitians</u>, homosexuals, <u>hemophiliacs</u>, and heroin users.[185] In the general press, the term "GRID", which stood for <u>gay-related immune deficiency</u>, had been coined.[186] However, after determining that AIDS was not isolated to the <u>gay community</u>,[184] it was realized that the term GRID was misleading and the term AIDS was introduced at a meeting in July 1982.[187] By September 1982 the CDC started referring to the disease as AIDS.[188]

In 1983, two separate research groups led by <u>Robert Gallo</u> and <u>Luc Montagnier</u> independently declared that a novel retrovirus may have been infecting people with AIDS, and published their findings in the same issue of the journal *Science*.[189][190] Gallo claimed that a virus his group had isolated from a person with AIDS was strikingly similar in <u>shape</u> to other <u>human T-lymphotropic viruses</u> (HTLVs) his group had been the first to isolate. Gallo's group called their newly isolated virus HTLV-III. At the same time, Montagnier's group isolated a virus from a person presenting with swelling of the <u>lymph nodes</u> of the neck and <u>physical weakness</u>, two characteristic symptoms of AIDS. Contradicting the report from Gallo's group, Montagnier and his colleagues showed that core proteins of this virus were immunologically different from those of HTLV-I. Montagnier's group named their isolated virus lymphadenopathy-associated virus (LAV).[181] As these two viruses turned out to be the same, in 1986, LAV and HTLV-III were renamed HIV.[191]

Origins

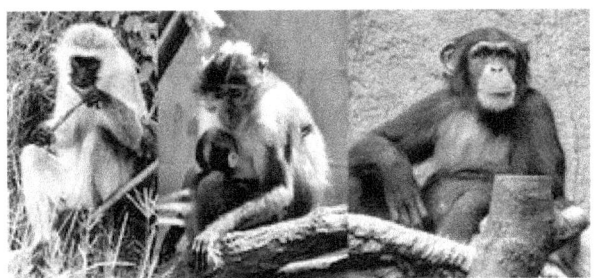

⌂

Left to right: the African green monkey source of SIV, the sooty mangabey source of HIV-2 and the chimpanzee source of HIV-1

Both HIV-1 and HIV-2 are believed to have originated in non-human primates in West-central Africa and were transferred to humans in the early 20th century.[5] HIV-1 appears to have originated in southern Cameroon through the evolution of SIV(cpz), a simian immunodeficiency virus (SIV) that infects wild chimpanzees (HIV-1 descends from the SIVcpz endemic in the chimpanzee subspecies *Pan troglodytes troglodytes*).[192][193] The closest relative of HIV-2 is SIV(smm), a virus of the sooty mangabey (*Cercocebus atys atys*), an Old World monkey living in coastal West Africa (from southern Senegal to western Côte d'Ivoire).[66] New World monkeys such as the owl monkey are resistant to HIV-1 infection, possibly because of a genomic fusion of two viral resistance genes.[194] HIV-1 is thought to have jumped the species barrier on at least three separate occasions, giving rise to the three groups of the virus, M, N, and O.[195]

There is evidence that humans who participate in bushmeat activities, either as hunters or as bushmeat vendors, commonly acquire SIV.[196] However, SIV is a weak virus which is typically suppressed by the human immune system within weeks of infection. It is thought that several transmissions of the virus from individual to individual in quick succession are necessary to allow it enough time to mutate into HIV.[197] Furthermore, due to its relatively low person-to-person transmission rate, SIV can only spread throughout the population in the presence of one or more high-risk transmission channels, which are thought to have been absent in Africa before the 20th century.

Specific proposed high-risk transmission channels, allowing the virus to adapt to humans and spread throughout the society, depend on the proposed timing of the animal-to-human crossing. Genetic studies of the virus suggest that the most recent common ancestor of the HIV-1 M group dates back to circa 1910.[198] Proponents of this dating link the HIV epidemic with the emergence of colonialism and growth of large colonial African cities, leading to social changes, including a higher degree of sexual promiscuity, the spread of prostitution, and the accompanying high frequency of genital ulcer diseases (such as syphilis) in nascent colonial cities.[199] While transmission rates of HIV during vaginal intercourse are low under regular circumstances, they are increased many fold if one of the partners suffers from a sexually transmitted infection causing genital ulcers. Early 1900s colonial cities were notable due to their high prevalence of prostitution and genital ulcers, to the degree that, as of 1928, as many as 45% of female residents of eastern Kinshasa were thought to have been prostitutes, and, as of 1933, around 15% of all residents of the same city had syphilis.[199]

An alternative view holds that unsafe medical practices in Africa after World War II, such as unsterile reuse of single use syringes during mass vaccination, antibiotic and anti-malaria treatment campaigns, were the initial vector that allowed the virus to adapt to humans and spread.[197][200][201]

The earliest well documented case of HIV in human dates back to 1959 in the Congo.[202] The virus may have been present in the United States as early as 1966,[203] but the vast majority of infections occurring outside sub-Saharan Africa (including the U.S.) can be traced back to a single unknown individual who became infected with HIV in Haiti and then brought the infection to the United States sometime around 1969.[204] the epidemic then rapidly spread among high-risk groups (initially, sexually promiscuous men who have sex with men). By 1978, the prevalence of HIV-1 among gay male residents of New York and San Francisco was estimated at 5%, suggesting that several thousand individuals in the country had been infected.[204]

Society and culture

Stigma

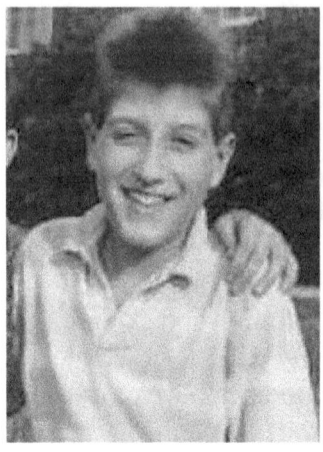

Ryan White became a poster child for HIV after being expelled from school because he was infected.
Main article: Discrimination against people with HIV/AIDS

AIDS stigma exists around the world in a variety of ways, including ostracism, rejection, discrimination and avoidance of HIV infected people; compulsory HIV testing without prior consent or protection of confidentiality; violence against HIV infected individuals or people who are perceived to be infected with HIV; and the quarantine of HIV infected individuals.[205] Stigma-related violence or the fear of violence prevents many people from seeking HIV testing, returning for their results, or securing treatment, possibly turning what could be a manageable chronic illness into a death sentence and perpetuating the spread of HIV.[206]

AIDS stigma has been further divided into the following three categories:

- *Instrumental AIDS stigma*—a reflection of the fear and apprehension that are likely to be associated with any deadly and transmissible illness.[207]
- *Symbolic AIDS stigma*—the use of HIV/AIDS to express attitudes toward the social groups or lifestyles perceived to be associated with the disease.[207]

- *Courtesy AIDS stigma*—stigmatization of people connected to the issue of HIV/AIDS or HIV-positive people.[208]

Often, AIDS stigma is expressed in conjunction with one or more other stigmas, particularly those associated with homosexuality, bisexuality, promiscuity, prostitution, and intravenous drug use.[209]

In many developed countries, there is an association between AIDS and homosexuality or bisexuality, and this association is correlated with higher levels of sexual prejudice, such as anti-homosexual/bisexual attitudes.[210] There is also a perceived association between AIDS and all male-male sexual behavior, including sex between uninfected men.[207] However, the dominant mode of spread worldwide for HIV remains heterosexual transmission.[211]

In 2003, as part of an overall reform of marriage and population legislation, it became legal for people with AIDS to marry in China.[212]

Economic impact

Main articles: Economic impact of HIV/AIDS and Cost of HIV treatment

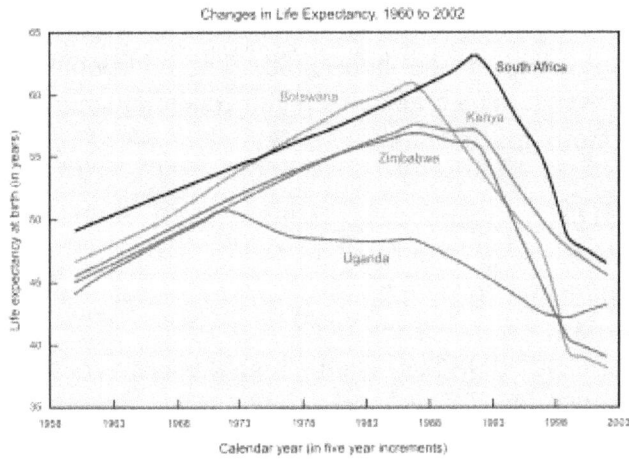

Changes in Life Expectancy, 1960 to 2002

Changes in life expectancy in some African countries

HIV/AIDS affects the economics of both individuals and countries.[171] The gross domestic product of the most affected countries has decreased due to the lack of human capital.[171][213] Without proper nutrition, health care and medicine, large numbers of people die from AIDS-related complications. They will not only be unable to work, but will also require significant medical care. It is estimated that as of 2007 there were 12 million AIDS orphans.[171] many are cared for by elderly grandparents.[214]

By affecting mainly young adults, AIDS reduces the taxable population, in turn reducing the resources available for public expenditures such as education and health services not related to AIDS resulting in increasing pressure for the state's finances and slower growth of the economy. This causes a slower growth of the tax base, an effect that is reinforced if there are growing expenditures on treating the sick, training (to replace sick workers), sick pay and caring for AIDS orphans. This is especially true if the sharp increase in adult mortality shifts the responsibility and blame from the family to the government in caring for these orphans.[214]

At the household level, AIDS causes both loss of income and increased spending on healthcare. A study in Côte d'Ivoire showed that households having a person with HIV/AIDS, spent twice as much on medical expenses as other households. This additional expenditure also leaves less income to spend on education and other personal or family investment.[215]

Religion and AIDS

Main article: Religion and HIV/AIDS

The topic of religion and AIDS has become highly controversial in the past twenty years, primarily because some religious authorities have publicly declared their opposition to the use of condoms.[216][217] The religious approach to prevent the spread of

AIDS according to a report by American health expert Matthew Hanley titled *The Catholic Church and the Global AIDS Crisis* argues that cultural changes are needed including a re-emphasis on fidelity within marriage and sexual abstinence outside of it.[217]

Some religious organisations have claimed that prayer can cure HIV/AIDS. In 2011, the BBC reported that some churches in London were claiming that prayer would cure AIDS, and the Hackney-based Centre for the Study of Sexual Health and HIV reported that several people stopped taking their medication, sometimes on the direct advice of their pastor, leading to a number of deaths.[218] The Synagogue Church Of All Nations advertise an "anointing water" to promote God's healing, although the group deny advising people to stop taking medication.[218]

Media portrayal

Main article: Media portrayal of HIV/AIDS

One of the first high-profile cases of AIDS was the American Rock Hudson, a gay actor who had been married and divorced earlier in life, who died on 2 October 1985 having announced that he was suffering from the virus on 25 July that year. He had been diagnosed during 1984.[219] A notable British casualty of AIDS that year was Nicholas Eden, a gay politician and son of the late prime minister Anthony Eden.[220] On November 24, 1991, the virus claimed the life of British rock star Freddie Mercury, lead singer of the band Queen, who died from an AIDS related illness having only revealed the diagnosis on the previous day.[221] However he had been diagnosed as HIV positive during 1987.[222] One of the first high-profile heterosexual cases of the virus was Arthur Ashe, the American tennis player. He was diagnosed as HIV positive on 31 August 1988, having contracted the virus from blood transfusions during heart surgery earlier in the 1980s. Further tests within 24 hours of the initial diagnosis revealed that Ashe had AIDS, but he did not tell the public about his diagnosis until April 1992.[223] He died, aged 49, as a result on 6 February 1993.[224]

Therese Frare's photograph of gay activist <u>David Kirby</u>, as he lay dying from AIDS while surrounded by family, was taken in April 1990. *LIFE magazine* said the photo became the one image "most powerfully identified with the HIV/AIDS epidemic." The photo was displayed in *LIFE magazine*, was the winner of the <u>World Press Photo</u>, and acquired worldwide notoriety after being used in a <u>United Colors of Benetton</u> advertising campaign in 1992.[225] In 1996, <u>Johnson Aziga</u> a Ugandan-born Canadian was diagnosed with HIV, but subsequently had unprotected sex with 11 women without disclosing his diagnosis. By 2003 seven had contracted HIV, and two died from complications related to AIDS.[226][227] Aziga was convicted of <u>first-degree murder</u> and is liable to a life sentence.[228]

Denial, conspiracies

Main articles: <u>AIDS denialism</u> and <u>Discredited HIV/AIDS origins theories</u>

A small group of individuals continue to dispute the connection between HIV and AIDS,[229] the existence of HIV itself, or the validity of HIV testing and treatment methods.[230][231] These claims, known as AIDS denialism, have been examined and rejected by the scientific community.[232] However, they have had a significant political impact, particularly <u>in South Africa</u>, where the government's official embrace of AIDS denialism (1999–2005) was responsible for its ineffective response to that country's AIDS epidemic, and has been blamed for hundreds of thousands of avoidable deaths and HIV infections.[233][234][235]

Several discredited <u>conspiracy theories</u> have held that HIV was created by scientists, either inadvertently or deliberately. <u>Operation INFEKTION</u> was a worldwide Soviet <u>active measures</u> operation to spread the claim that the United States had created HIV/AIDS. Surveys show that a significant number of people believed – and continue to believe – in such claims.[236]

Misconceptions

Main article: Misconceptions about HIV/AIDS

There are many misconceptions about HIV and AIDS. Three of the most common are that AIDS can spread through casual contact, that sexual intercourse with a virgin will cure AIDS,[237][238][239] and that HIV can infect only homosexual men and drug users. Other misconceptions are that any act of anal intercourse between two uninfected gay men can lead to HIV infection, and that open discussion of HIV and homosexuality in schools will lead to increased rates of AIDS.[240][241]

Research

Main article: HIV/AIDS research

HIV/AIDS research includes all medical research which attempts to prevent, treat, or cure HIV/AIDS along with fundamental research about the nature of HIV as an infectious agent and AIDS as the disease caused by HIV.

Many governments and research institutions participate in HIV/AIDS research. This research includes behavioral health interventions such as sex education, and drug development, such as research into microbicides for sexually transmitted diseases, HIV vaccines, and antiretroviral drugs. Other medical research areas include the topics of pre-exposure prophylaxis, post-exposure prophylaxis, and circumcision and HIV.

References

Notes

1.   **Jump up** ^ Sepkowitz KA (June 2001). "AIDS—the first 20 years". *N. Engl. J. Med.* **344** (23): 1764–72. doi:10.1056/NEJM200106073442306. PMID 11396444.
2.   ^ Jump up to: *a b c d e f g h i j* Markowitz, edited by William N. Rom ; associate editor, Steven B. (2007). *Environmental and occupational medicine* (4th ed.). Philadelphia: Wolters

Kluwer/Lippincott Williams & Wilkins. p. 745. ISBN 978-0-7817-6299-1.

3.   **Jump up** ^ "HIV and Its Transmission". Centers for Disease Control and Prevention. 2003. Archived from the original on February 4, 2005. Retrieved May 23, 2006.

4.   ^ Jump up to: *a b* UNAIDS, WHO (December 2007). "2007 AIDS epidemic update" (PDF). Retrieved 2008-03-12.

5.   ^ Jump up to: *a b* Sharp, PM; Hahn, BH (September 2011). "Origins of HIV and the AIDS Pandemic". *Cold Spring Harbor perspectives in medicine* **1** (1): a006841. doi:10.1101/cshperspect.a006841. PMC 3234451. PMID 22229120.

6.   **Jump up** ^ Gallo RC (2006). "A reflection on HIV/AIDS research after 25 years". *Retrovirology* **3**: 72. doi:10.1186/1742-4690-3-72. PMC 1629027. PMID 17054781.

7.   ^ Jump up to: *a b* "Fact Sheet". *UNAIDS.org*. 2013. Retrieved December 4, 2013.

8.   ^ Jump up to: *a b* Kallings LO (2008). "The first postmodern pandemic: 25 years of HIV/AIDS". *Journal of Internal Medicine* **263** (3): 218–43. doi:10.1111/j.1365-2796.2007.01910.x. PMID 18205765.(subscription required)

9.   **Jump up** ^ Harden, Victoria Angela (2012). *AIDS at 30: A History*. Potomac Books Inc. p. 324. ISBN 1-59797-294-0.

10.   ^ Jump up to: *a b c d e f* Mandell, Bennett, and Dolan (2010). Chapter 121.

11.   ^ Jump up to: *a b c* "Stages of HIV". *U.S. Department of Health & Human Services*. Dec 2010. Retrieved 13 June 2012.

12.   ^ Jump up to: *a b c d e f g h i j k l m n o p* WHO case definitions of *HIV for surveillance and revised clinical staging and immunological classification of HIV-related disease in adults and children.* (PDF). Geneva: World Health Organization. 2007. pp. 6–16. ISBN 978-92-4-159562-9.

13.   **Jump up** ^ *Diseases and disorders.*. Tarrytown, NY: Marshall Cavendish. 2008. p. 25. ISBN 978-0-7614-7771-6.

14.   ^ Jump up to: *a b c d e f g h i j k l m n* Mandell, Bennett, and Dolan (2010). Chapter 118.

15.   ^ Jump up to: *a b c d e f g h i j k l m n o p q r* Vogel, M; Schwarze-Zander, C; Wasmuth, JC; Spengler, U; Sauerbruch, T; Rockstroh, JK (July 2010). "The treatment of patients with HIV". *Deutsches Ärzteblatt international* **107** (28–29): 507–15; quiz 516. doi:10.3238/arztebl.2010.0507. PMC 2915483. PMID 20703338.

16.   **Jump up** ^ Evian, Clive (2006). *Primary HIV/AIDS care: a practical guide for primary health care personnel in a clinical and supportive setting* (Updated 4th ed.). Houghton [South Africa]: Jacana. p. 29. ISBN 978-1-77009-198-6.

17.   **Jump up** ^ *Radiology of AIDS*. Berlin [u.a.]: Springer. 2001. p. 19. ISBN 978-3-540-66510-6.

18.   **Jump up** ^ Elliott, Tom (2012). *Lecture Notes: Medical Microbiology and Infection.* John Wiley & Sons. p. 273. ISBN 978-1-118-37226-5.

19.   ^ Jump up to: *a b* Blankson, JN (March 2010). "Control of HIV-1 replication in elite suppressors". *Discovery medicine* **9** (46): 261–6. PMID 20350494.

20.   **Jump up** ^ Walker, BD (Aug–Sep 2007). "Elite control of HIV Infection: implications for vaccines and treatment". *Topics in HIV medicine : a publication of the International AIDS Society, USA* **15** (4): 134–6. PMID 17720999.

21.   **Jump up** ^ Holmes CB, Losina E, Walensky RP, Yazdanpanah Y, Freedberg KA (2003). "Review of human immunodeficiency virus type 1-related opportunistic infections in sub-Saharan Africa". *Clin. Infect. Dis.* **36** (5): 656–662. doi:10.1086/367655. PMID 12594648.

22.   **Jump up** ^ Chu, C; Selwyn, PA (2011-02-15). "Complications of HIV infection: a systems-based approach". *American family physician* **83** (4): 395–406. PMID 21322514.

23.   ^ Jump up to: *a b c d e* Mandell, Bennett, and Dolan (2010). Chapter 169.

24.   **Jump up** ^ "AIDS". *MedlinePlus*. A.D.A.M. Retrieved 14 June 2012.

25.   **Jump up** ^ Sestak K (July 2005). "Chronic diarrhea and AIDS: insights into studies with non-human primates". *Curr. HIV Res.* **3** (3): 199–205. doi:10.2174/1570162054368084. PMID 16022653.

26.   **Jump up** ^ Murray ED, Buttner N, Price BH (2012). "Depression and Psychosis in Neurological Practice". In Bradley WG, Daroff RB, Fenichel GM, Jankovic J. *Bradley's Neurology in Clinical Practice: Expert Consult - Online and Print, 6e (Bradley, Neurology in Clinical Practice e-dition 2v Set)* **1** (6th ed.). Philadelphia, PA: Elsevier/Saunders. p. 101. ISBN 1-4377-0434-4.

27.   ^ Jump up to: *a b* Smith, DK; Grohskopf, LA; Black, RJ; Auerbach, JD; Veronese, F; Struble, KA; Cheever, L; Johnson, M; Paxton, LA; Onorato, IM; Greenberg, AE; U.S. Department of Health and Human, Services (21 January 2005). "Antiretroviral postexposure prophylaxis after sexual, injection-drug use, or other nonoccupational exposure to HIV in the United States: recommendations from the U.S. Department of Health and Human Services.". *MMWR. Recommendations and reports : Morbidity and mortality weekly report. Recommendations and reports / Centers for Disease Control* **54** (RR-2): 1–20. PMID 15660015.

28.   **Jump up** ^ Coovadia H (2004). "Antiretroviral agents—how best to protect infants from HIV and save their mothers from AIDS". *N. Engl. J. Med.* **351** (3): 289–292. doi:10.1056/NEJMe048128. PMID 15247337.

29.   ^ Jump up to: *a b c d* Kripke, C (1 August 2007). "Antiretroviral prophylaxis for occupational exposure to HIV.". *American family physician* **76** (3): 375–6. PMID 17708137.

30.   ^ Jump up to: *a b c d* Dosekun, O; Fox, J (July 2010). "An overview of the relative risks of different sexual behaviours on HIV transmission.". *Current opinion in HIV and AIDS* **5** (4): 291–7. doi:10.1097/COH.0b013e32833a88a3. PMID 20543603.

31.   **Jump up ^** Cunha, Burke (2012). *Antibiotic Essentials 2012* (11 ed.). Jones & Bartlett Publishers. p. 303. ISBN 9781449693831.

32.   ^ Jump up to: *a b* Boily, MC; Baggaley, RF; Wang, L; Masse, B; White, RG; Hayes, RJ; Alary, M (February 2009). "Heterosexual risk of HIV-1 infection per sexual act: systematic review and meta-analysis of observational studies.". *The Lancet infectious diseases* **9** (2): 118–29. doi:10.1016/S1473-3099(09)70021-0. PMID 19179227.

33.   **Jump up ^** Baggaley, RF; White, RG; Boily, MC (December 2008). "Systematic review of orogenital HIV-1 transmission probabilities.". *International Journal of Epidemiology* **37** (6): 1255–65. doi:10.1093/ije/dyn151. PMC 2638872. PMID 18664564.

34.   **Jump up ^** van der Kuyl, AC; Cornelissen, M (2007-09-24). "Identifying HIV-1 dual infections". *Retrovirology* **4**: 67. doi:10.1186/1742-4690-4-67. PMC 2045676. PMID 17892568.

35.   ^ Jump up to: *a b* "HIV in the United States: An Overview". *Center for Disease Control and Prevention*. March 2012.

36.   ^ Jump up to: *a b c d e f g* Boily MC, Baggaley RF, Wang L, Masse B, White RG, Hayes RJ, Alary M (February 2009). "Heterosexual risk of HIV-1 infection per sexual act: systematic review and meta-analysis of observational studies". *The Lancet Infectious Diseases* **9** (2): 118–129. doi:10.1016/S1473-3099(09)70021-0. PMID 19179227.

37.   **Jump up ^** Beyrer, C; Baral, SD; van Griensven, F; Goodreau, SM; Chariyalertsak, S; Wirtz, AL; Brookmeyer, R (Jul 28, 2012). "Global epidemiology of HIV infection in men who have sex with men". *Lancet* **380** (9839): 367–77. doi:10.1016/S0140-6736(12)60821-6. PMID 22819660.

38.   **Jump up ^** Yu, M; Vajdy, M (August 2010). "Mucosal HIV transmission and vaccination strategies through oral compared with vaginal and rectal routes". *Expert opinion on biological therapy* **10** (8): 1181–95. doi:10.1517/14712598.2010.496776. PMC 2904634. PMID 20624114.

39.   **Jump up ^** Stürchler, Dieter A. (2006). *Exposure a guide to sources of infections*. Washington, DC: ASM Press. p. 544. ISBN 9781555813765.

40.   **Jump up ^** al.], edited by Richard Pattman (2010). *Oxford handbook of genitourinary medicine, HIV, and sexual health* (2nd ed.). Oxford: Oxford University Press. p. 95. ISBN 9780199571666.

41.   ^ Jump up to: *a b c* Dosekun, O; Fox, J (July 2010). "An overview of the relative risks of different sexual behaviours on HIV transmission". *Current Opinion in HIV and AIDS* **5** (4): 291–7. doi:10.1097/COH.0b013e32833a88a3. PMID 20543603.

42.   ^ Jump up to: *a b* Ng, BE; Butler, LM; Horvath, T; Rutherford, GW (2011-03-16). "Population-based biomedical sexually transmitted infection control interventions for reducing HIV infection". In Butler, Lisa M. *Cochrane database of systematic reviews (Online)* (3): CD001220. doi:10.1002/14651858.CD001220.pub3. PMID 21412869.

43.   **Jump up ^** Anderson, J (February 2012). "Women and HIV: motherhood and more". *Current Opinion in Infectious Diseases* **25** (1): 58–65. doi:10.1097/QCO.0b013e32834ef514. PMID 22156896.

44.   **Jump up ^** Kerrigan, Deanna (2012). *The Global HIV Epidemics among Sex Workers*. World Bank Publications. p. 1. ISBN 9780821397756.

45.   **Jump up ^** Aral, Sevgi (2013). *The New Public Health and STD/HIV Prevention: Personal, Public and Health Systems Approaches*. Springer. p. 120. ISBN 9781461445265.

46.   **Jump up ^** Klimas, N; Koneru, AO; Fletcher, MA (June 2008). "Overview of HIV". *Psychosomatic Medicine* **70** (5): 523–30. doi:10.1097/PSY.0b013e31817ae69f. PMID 18541903.

47.   **Jump up ^** Draughon, JE; Sheridan, DJ (2012). "Nonoccupational post exposure prophylaxis following sexual assault in industrialized low-HIV-prevalence countries: a review". *Psychology, health & medicine* **17** (2): 235–54. doi:10.1080/13548506.2011.579984. PMID 22372741.

48.   ^ Jump up to: *a b* Baggaley, RF; Boily, MC; White, RG; Alary, M (2006-04-04). "Risk of HIV-1 transmission for parenteral exposure and blood transfusion: a systematic review and meta-analysis". *AIDS (London, England)* **20** (6): 805–12. doi:10.1097/01.aids.0000218543.46963.6d. PMID 16549963.

49.   **Jump up ^** "Will I need a blood transfusion?". *NHS patient information*. National Health Services. 2011. Retrieved August 29, 2012.

50.   **Jump up ^** UNAIDS 2011 pg. 60–70

51.   **Jump up ^** "Blood safety ... for too few". WHO. 2001. Retrieved January 17, 2006.

52.   ^ Jump up to: *a b c* Reid, SR (2009-08-28). "Injection drug use, unsafe medical injections, and HIV in Africa: a systematic review". *Harm reduction journal* **6**: 24. doi:10.1186/1477-7517-6-24. PMC 2741434. PMID 19715601.

53.   ^ Jump up to: *a b* "Basic Information about HIV and AIDS". *Center for Disease Control and Prevention*. April 2012.

54.   **Jump up ^** Crans, Wayne J. (June 1, 2010). "Why Mosquitoes Cannot Transmit AIDS". *rci.rutgers.edu*. Rutgers University. New Jersey Agricultural Experiment Station Publication

No. H-40101-01-93. Archived from the original on March 29, 2014. Retrieved March 29, 2014.

55.　　　　^ Jump up to: *a b c d e f* Coutsoudis, A; Kwaan, L; Thomson, M (October 2010). "Prevention of vertical transmission of HIV-1 in resource-limited settings". *Expert review of anti-infective therapy* **8** (10): 1163–75. doi:10.1586/eri.10.94. PMID 20954881.

56.　　　　**Jump up** ^ "Fluids of transmission". *AIDS.gov*. United States Department of Health and Human Services. 1 November 2011. Retrieved 14 September 2012.

57.　　　　^ Jump up to: *a b* Thorne, C; Newell, ML (June 2007). "HIV". *Seminars in fetal & neonatal medicine* **12** (3): 174–81. doi:10.1016/j.siny.2007.01.009. PMID 17321814.

58.　　　　**Jump up** ^ Alimonti JB, Ball TB, Fowke KR (2003). "Mechanisms of CD4+ T lymphocyte cell death in human immunodeficiency virus infection and AIDS". *J. Gen. Virol.* **84** (7): 1649–1661. doi:10.1099/vir.0.19110-0. PMID 12810858.

59.　　　　**Jump up** ^ International Committee on Taxonomy of Viruses (2002). "61.0.6. Lentivirus". National Institutes of Health. Archived from the original on 2006-04-18. Retrieved 2012-06-25.

60.　　　　**Jump up** ^ International Committee on Taxonomy of Viruses (2002). "61. Retroviridae". National Institutes of Health. Archived from the original on 2006-06-29. Retrieved 2012-06-25.

61.　　　　**Jump up** ^ Lévy, J. A. (1993). "HIV pathogenesis and long-term survival". *AIDS* **7** (11): 1401–10. doi:10.1097/00002030-199311000-00001. PMID 8280406.

62.　　　　**Jump up** ^ Smith, Johanna A.; Daniel, René (Division of Infectious Diseases, Center for Human Virology, Thomas Jefferson University, Philadelphia) (2006). "Following the path of the virus: the exploitation of host DNA repair mechanisms by retroviruses". *ACS Chem Biol* **1** (4): 217–26. doi:10.1021/cb600131q. PMID 17163676.

63.　　　　**Jump up** ^ Martínez, edited by Miguel Angel (2010). *RNA interference and viruses : current innovations and future trends*. Norfolk: Caister Academic Press. p. 73. ISBN 9781904455561.

64.　　　　**Jump up** ^ *Immunology, infection, and immunity*. Washington, D.C.: ASM Press. 2004. p. 550. ISBN 9781555812461.

65.　　　　**Jump up** ^ Gilbert, PB et al. (28 February 2003). "Comparison of HIV-1 and HIV-2 infectivity from a prospective cohort study in Senegal". *Statistics in Medicine* **22** (4): 573–593. doi:10.1002/sim.1342. PMID 12590415.

66.　　　　^ Jump up to: *a b* Reeves, J. D. and Doms, R. W (2002). "Human Immunodeficiency Virus Type 2". *J. Gen. Virol.* **83** (Pt 6): 1253–65. doi:10.1099/vir.0.18253-0. PMID 12029140.

67.　　　　**Jump up** ^ Piatak, M., Jr, Saag, M. S., Yang, L. C., Clark, S. J., Kappes, J. C., Luk, K. C., Hahn, B. H., Shaw, G. M. and Lifson, J.D. (1993). "High levels of HIV-1 in plasma during all stages of infection determined by competitive PCR". *Science* **259** (5102): 1749–1754.

Bibcode:1993Sci...259.1749P. doi:10.1126/science.8096089. PMID 8096089.

68.   **Jump up** ^ Pantaleo G, Demarest JF, Schacker T, Vaccarezza M, Cohen OJ, Daucher M, Graziosi C, Schnittman SS, Quinn TC, Shaw GM, Perrin L, Tambussi G, Lazzarin A, Sekaly RP, Soudeyns H, Corey L, Fauci AS. (1997). "The qualitative nature of the primary immune response to HIV infection is a prognosticator of disease progression independent of the initial level of plasma viremia". *Proc Natl Acad Sci U S A.* **94** (1): 254–258. Bibcode:1997PNAS...94..254P. doi:10.1073/pnas.94.1.254. PMC 19306. PMID 8990195.

69.   **Jump up** ^ Hel Z, McGhee JR, Mestecky J (June 2006). "HIV infection: first battle decides the war". *Trends Immunol.* **27** (6): 274–81. doi:10.1016/j.it.2006.04.007. PMID 16679064.

70.   **Jump up** ^ Arie J. Zuckerman et al. (eds) (2007). *Principles and practice of clinical virology* (6th ed.). Hoboken, N.J.: Wiley. p. 905. ISBN 978-0-470-51799-4.

71.   **Jump up** ^ Mehandru S, Poles MA, Tenner-Racz K, Horowitz A, Hurley A, Hogan C, Boden D, Racz P, Markowitz M (September 2004). "Primary HIV-1 infection is associated with preferential depletion of CD4+ T cells from effector sites in the gastrointestinal tract". *J. Exp. Med.* **200** (6): 761–70. doi:10.1084/jem.20041196. PMC 2211967. PMID 15365095.

72.   **Jump up** ^ Brenchley JM, Schacker TW, Ruff LE, Price DA, Taylor JH, Beilman GJ, Nguyen PL, Khoruts A, Larson M, Haase AT, Douek DC (September 2004). "CD4+ T cell depletion during all stages of HIV disease occurs predominantly in the gastrointestinal tract". *J. Exp. Med.* **200** (6): 749–59. doi:10.1084/jem.20040874. PMC 2211962. PMID 15365096.

73.   **Jump up** ^ Olson, WC; Jacobson, JM (March 2009). "CCR5 monoclonal antibodies for HIV-1 therapy.". *Current opinion in HIV and AIDS* **4** (2): 104–11. doi:10.1097/COH.0b013e3283224015. PMID 19339948.

74.   ^ Jump up to: [a] [b] editor, Julio Aliberti, (2011). *Control of Innate and Adaptive Immune Responses During Infectious Diseases.*. New York, NY: Springer Verlag. p. 145. ISBN 978-1-4614-0483-5.

75.   **Jump up** ^ Appay V, Sauce D (January 2008). "Immune activation and inflammation in HIV-1 infection: causes and consequences". *J. Pathol.* **214** (2): 231–41. doi:10.1002/path.2276. PMID 18161758.

76.   **Jump up** ^ Brenchley JM, Price DA, Schacker TW, Asher TE, Silvestri G, Rao S, Kazzaz Z, Bornstein E, Lambotte O, Altmann D, Blazar BR, Rodriguez B, Teixeira-Johnson L, Landay A, Martin JN, Hecht FM, Picker LJ, Lederman MM, Deeks SG, Douek DC (December 2006). "Microbial translocation is a cause of systemic immune activation in chronic HIV infection". *Nat. Med.* **12** (12): 1365–71. doi:10.1038/nm1511. PMID 17115046.

77.   **Jump up** ^ Moyer,, Virginia A. (April 2013). "Screening for HIV: U.S. Preventive Services Task Force Recommendation Statement". *Annals of Internal Medicine*. doi:10.7326/0003-4819-159-1-201307020-00645.

78.   ^ Jump up to: *a b* Kellerman, S; Essajee, S (Jul 20, 2010). "HIV testing for children in resource-limited settings: what are we waiting for?". *PLoS medicine* **7** (7): e1000285. doi:10.1371/journal.pmed.1000285. PMC 2907270. PMID 20652012.

79.   ^ Jump up to: *a b c* UNAIDS 2011 pg. 70–80

80.   ^ Jump up to: *a b c d* Schneider, E; Whitmore, S; Glynn, KM; Dominguez, K; Mitsch, A; McKenna, MT; Centers for Disease Control and Prevention, (CDC) (2008-12-05). "Revised surveillance case definitions for HIV infection among adults, adolescents, and children aged <18 months and for HIV infection and AIDS among children aged 18 months to <13 years--United States, 2008". *MMWR. Recommendations and reports : Morbidity and mortality weekly report. Recommendations and reports / Centers for Disease Control* **57** (RR–10): 1–12. PMID 19052530.

81.   **Jump up** ^ Crosby, R; Bounse, S (March 2012). "Condom effectiveness: where are we now?". *Sexual health* **9** (1): 10–7. doi:10.1071/SH11036. PMID 22348628.

82.   **Jump up** ^ "Condom Facts and Figures". WHO. August 2003. Retrieved January 17, 2006.

83.   **Jump up** ^ Gallo, MF; Kilbourne-Brook, M; Coffey, PS (March 2012). "A review of the effectiveness and acceptability of the female condom for dual protection". *Sexual health* **9** (1): 18–26. doi:10.1071/SH11037. PMID 22348629.

84.   ^ Jump up to: *a b* Celum, C; Baeten, JM (February 2012). "Tenofovir-based pre-exposure prophylaxis for HIV prevention: evolving evidence". *Current Opinion in Infectious Diseases* **25** (1): 51–7. doi:10.1097/QCO.0b013e32834ef5ef. PMC 3266126. PMID 22156901.

85.   **Jump up** ^ Baptista, M; Ramalho-Santos, J (2009-11-01). "Spermicides, microbicides and antiviral agents: recent advances in the development of novel multi-functional compounds". *Mini reviews in medicinal chemistry* **9** (13): 1556–67. doi:10.2174/138955709790361548. PMID 20205637.

86.   **Jump up** ^ Siegfried, N; Muller, M; Deeks, JJ; Volmink, J (2009-04-15). "Male circumcision for prevention of heterosexual acquisition of HIV in men". In Siegfried, Nandi. *Cochrane database of systematic reviews (Online)* (2): CD003362. doi:10.1002/14651858.CD003362.pub2. PMID 19370585.

87.   **Jump up** ^ "WHO and UNAIDS announce recommendations from expert consultation on male circumcision for HIV prevention". World Health Organization. Mar 28, 2007.

88.   **Jump up** ^ Larke, N (2010 May 27 – Jun 9). "Male circumcision, HIV and sexually transmitted infections: a review". *British journal of nursing (Mark Allen Publishing)* **19** (10): 629–34. PMID 20622758.

89.   **Jump up** ^ Eaton, L; Kalichman, SC (November 2009). "Behavioral aspects of male circumcision for the prevention of HIV infection". *Current HIV/AIDS reports* **6** (4): 187–93. doi:10.1007/s11904-009-0025-9. PMC 3557929. PMID 19849961.(subscription required)

90.   **Jump up** ^ Kim, HH; Li, PS, Goldstein, M (November 2010). "Male circumcision: Africa and beyond?". *Current Opinion in Urology* **20** (6): 515–9. doi:10.1097/MOU.0b013e32833f1b21. PMID 20844437.

91.   **Jump up** ^ Templeton, DJ; Millett, GA, Grulich, AE (February 2010). "Male circumcision to reduce the risk of HIV and sexually transmitted infections among men who have sex with men". *Current Opinion in Infectious Diseases* **23** (1): 45–52. doi:10.1097/QCO.0b013e328334e54d. PMID 19935420.

92.   **Jump up** ^ Wiysonge, Charles Shey; Kongnyuy, Eugene J; Shey, Muki; Muula, Adamson S; Navti, Osric B; Akl, Elie A; Lo, Ying-Ru (June 15, 2011). "Male circumcision for prevention of homosexual acquisition of HIV in men". In Wiysonge, Charles Shey. *Cochrane Database of Systematic Reviews* (John Wiley & Sons, Ltd) (6): CD007496. doi:10.1002/14651858.CD007496.pub2. PMID 21678366.

93.   **Jump up** ^ Eaton LA, Kalichman S (December 2007). "Risk compensation in HIV prevention: implications for vaccines, microbicides, and other biomedical HIV prevention technologies". *Curr HIV/AIDS Rep* **4** (4): 165–72. doi:10.1007/s11904-007-0024-7. PMC 2937204. PMID 18366947.

94.   **Jump up** ^ Underhill K, Operario D, Montgomery P (2008). "Abstinence-only programs for HIV infection prevention in high-income countries". In Operario, Don. *Cochrane Database of Systematic Reviews* (4): CD005421. doi:10.1002/14651858.CD005421.pub2. PMID 17943855.

95.   **Jump up** ^ Tolli, MV (2012-05-28). "Effectiveness of peer education interventions for HIV prevention, adolescent pregnancy prevention and sexual health promotion for young people: a systematic review of European studies". *Health education research* **27** (5): 904–13. doi:10.1093/her/cys055. PMID 22641791.

96.   **Jump up** ^ Ljubojević, S; Lipozenčić, J (2010). "Sexually transmitted infections and adolescence". *Acta dermatovenerologica Croatica : ADC* **18** (4): 305–10. PMID 21251451.

97.   **Jump up** ^ Patel VL, Yoskowitz NA, Kaufman DR, Shortliffe EH (2008). "Discerning patterns of human immunodeficiency virus risk

in healthy young adults". *Am J Med* **121** (4): 758–764. doi:10.1016/j.amjmed.2008.04.022. PMC 2597652. PMID 18724961.

98.   **Jump up** ^ Anglemyer, A; Rutherford, GW; Baggaley, RC; Egger, M; Siegfried, N (2011-08-10). "Antiretroviral therapy for prevention of HIV transmission in HIV-discordant couples". In Rutherford, George W. *Cochrane database of systematic reviews (Online)* (8): CD009153. doi:10.1002/14651858.CD009153.pub2. PMID 21833973.

99.   **Jump up** ^ Chou R, Selph S, Dana T, et al. (November 2012). "Screening for HIV: systematic review to update the 2005 U.S. Preventive Services Task Force recommendation". *Annals of Internal Medicine* **157** (10): 706–18. doi:10.7326/0003-4819-157-10-201211200-00007. PMID 23165662.

100.   **Jump up** ^ Choopanya, Kachit; Martin, Michael; Suntharasamai, Pravan; Sangkum, Udomsak; Mock, Philip A; Leethochawalit, Manoj; Chiamwongpaet, Sithisat; Kitisin, Praphan; Natrujirote, Pitinan; Kittimunkong, Somyot; Chuachoowong, Rutt; Gvetadze, Roman J; McNicholl, Janet M; Paxton, Lynn A; Curlin, Marcel E; Hendrix, Craig W; Vanichseni, Suphak (1 June 2013). "Antiretroviral prophylaxis for HIV infection in injecting drug users in Bangkok, Thailand (the Bangkok Tenofovir Study): a randomised, double-blind, placebo-controlled phase 3 trial". *The Lancet* **381** (9883): 2083–2090. doi:10.1016/S0140-6736(13)61127-7.

101.   **Jump up** ^ Centers for Disease Control (CDC) (August 1987). "Recommendations for prevention of HIV transmission in health-care settings". *MMWR* **36** (Suppl 2): 1S–18S. PMID 3112554.

102.   ^ Jump up to: *ᵃ ᵇ* Kurth, AE; Celum, C; Baeten, JM; Vermund, SH; Wasserheit, JN (March 2011). "Combination HIV prevention: significance, challenges, and opportunities". *Current HIV/AIDS reports* **8** (1): 62–72. doi:10.1007/s11904-010-0063-3. PMC 3036787. PMID 20941553.

103.   **Jump up** ^ MacArthur, G. J.; Minozzi, S.; Martin, N.; Vickerman, P.; Deren, S.; Bruneau, J.; Degenhardt, L.; Hickman, M. (4 October 2012). "Opiate substitution treatment and HIV transmission in people who inject drugs: systematic review and meta-analysis". *BMJ* **345** (oct03 3): e5945–e5945. doi:10.1136/bmj.e5945.

104.   ^ Jump up to: *ᵃ ᵇ* [No authors listed] (April 2012). "HIV exposure through contact with body fluids". *Prescrire Int* **21** (126): 100–1, 103–5. PMID 22515138.

105.   **Jump up** ^ Kuhar DT, Henderson DK, Struble KA, et al. (September 2013). "Updated US Public Health Service Guidelines for the Management of Occupational Exposures to Human Immunodeficiency Virus and Recommendations for Postexposure Prophylaxis". *Infect Control Hosp Epidemiol* **34** (9): 875–92. doi:10.1086/672271. PMID 23917901.

106.   **Jump up** ^ Linden, JA (2011-09-01). "Clinical practice. Care of the adult patient after sexual assault". *The New England Journal of Medicine* **365** (9): 834–41. doi:10.1056/NEJMcp1102869. PMID 21879901.

107.   **Jump up** ^ Young, TN; Arens, FJ; Kennedy, GE; Laurie, JW; Rutherford, G (2007-01-24). "Antiretroviral post-exposure prophylaxis (PEP) for occupational HIV exposure". In Young, Taryn. *Cochrane database of systematic reviews (Online)* (1): CD002835. doi:10.1002/14651858.CD002835.pub3. PMID 17253483.

108.   **Jump up** ^ Siegfried, N; van der Merwe, L; Brocklehurst, P; Sint, TT (2011-07-06). "Antiretrovirals for reducing the risk of mother-to-child transmission of HIV infection". In Siegfried, Nandi. *Cochrane database of systematic reviews (Online)* (7): CD003510. doi:10.1002/14651858.CD003510.pub3. PMID 21735394.

109.   **Jump up** ^ "WHO HIV and Infant Feeding Technical Consultation Held on behalf of the Inter-agency Task Team (IATT) on Prevention of HIV – Infections in Pregnant Women, Mothers and their Infants – Consensus statement" (PDF). October 25–27, 2006. Archived from the original on April 9, 2008. Retrieved March 12, 2008.

110.   **Jump up** ^ Horvath, T; Madi, BC; Iuppa, IM; Kennedy, GE; Rutherford, G; Read, JS (2009-01-21). "Interventions for preventing late postnatal mother-to-child transmission of HIV". In Horvath, Tara. *Cochrane database of systematic reviews (Online)* (1): CD006734. doi:10.1002/14651858.CD006734.pub2. PMID 19160297.

111.   **Jump up** ^ UNAIDS (May 18, 2012). "The quest for an HIV vaccine".

112.   **Jump up** ^ Reynell, L; Trkola, A (2012-03-02). "HIV vaccines: an attainable goal?". *Swiss medical weekly* **142**: w13535. doi:10.4414/smw.2012.13535. PMID 22389197.

113.   **Jump up** ^ U.S. Army Office of the Surgeon General (March 21, 2011). "HIV Vaccine Trial in Thai Adults". ClinicalTrials.gov. Retrieved June 28, 2011.

114.   **Jump up** ^ U.S. Army Office of the Surgeon General (June 2, 2010). "Follow up of Thai Adult Volunteers With Breakthrough HIV Infection After Participation in a Preventive HIV Vaccine Trial". ClinicalTrials.gov.

115.   **Jump up** ^ May, MT; Ingle, SM (December 2011). "Life expectancy of HIV-positive adults: a review". *Sexual health* **8** (4): 526–33. doi:10.1071/SH11046. PMID 22127039.

116.   ^ Jump up to: [a] [b] [c] [d] UNAIDS 2011 pg. 1–10

117.   ^ Jump up to: [a] [b] [c] [d] [e] *Antiretroviral therapy for HIV infection in adults and adolescents: recommendations for a public health approach*. World Health Organization. 2010. pp. 19–20. ISBN 978-92-4-159976-4.

118.   ^ Jump up to: *ᵃ ᵇ ᶜ Consolidated guidelines on the use of antiretroviral drugs for treating and preventing HIV infection*. World Health Organization. 2013. pp. 28–30. ISBN 9789241505727.

119.   **Jump up** ^ Sax, PE; Baden, LR (2009-04-30). "When to start antiretroviral therapy—ready when you are?". *The New England Journal of Medicine* 360 (18): 1897–9. doi:10.1056/NEJMe0902713. PMID 19339713.

120.   **Jump up** ^ Siegfried, N; Uthman, OA; Rutherford, GW (2010-03-17). "Optimal time for initiation of antiretroviral therapy in asymptomatic, HIV-infected, treatment-naive adults". In Siegfried, Nandi. *Cochrane database of systematic reviews (Online)* (3): CD008272. doi:10.1002/14651858.CD008272.pub2. PMID 20238364.

121.   **Jump up** ^ "Guidelines for the Use of Antiretroviral Agents in HIV-1-Infected Adults and Adolescents" (pdf). *Department of Health and Human Services*. Feb 12, 2013. p. i. Retrieved 3 January 2014.

122.   **Jump up** ^ When To Start, Consortium; Sterne, JA; May, M; Costagliola, D; de Wolf, F; Phillips, AN; Harris, R; Funk, MJ; Geskus, RB; Gill, J; Dabis, F; Miró, JM; Justice, AC; Ledergerber, B; Fätkenheuer, G; Hogg, RS; Monforte, AD; Saag, M; Smith, C; Staszewski, S; Egger, M; Cole, SR (2009-04-18). "Timing of initiation of antiretroviral therapy in AIDS-free HIV-1-infected patients: a collaborative analysis of 18 HIV cohort studies". *Lancet* 373 (9672): 1352–63. doi:10.1016/S0140-6736(09)60612-7. PMC 2670965. PMID 19361855.

123.   **Jump up** ^ Beard, J; Feeley, F; Rosen, S (November 2009). "Economic and quality of life outcomes of antiretroviral therapy for HIV/AIDS in developing countries: a systematic literature review". *AIDS care* 21 (11): 1343–56. doi:10.1080/09540120902889926. PMID 20024710.

124.   **Jump up** ^ Orrell, C (November 2005). "Antiretroviral adherence in a resource-poor setting". *Current HIV/AIDS reports* 2 (4): 171–6. doi:10.1007/s11904-005-0012-8. PMID 16343374.

125.   **Jump up** ^ Malta, M; Strathdee, SA; Magnanini, MM; Bastos, FI (August 2008). "Adherence to antiretroviral therapy for human immunodeficiency virus/acquired immune deficiency syndrome among drug users: a systematic review". *Addiction (Abingdon, England)* 103 (8): 1242–57. doi:10.1111/j.1360-0443.2008.02269.x. PMID 18855813.

126.   **Jump up** ^ Nachega, JB; Marconi, VC; van Zyl, GU; Gardner, EM; Preiser, W; Hong, SY; Mills, EJ; Gross, R (April 2011). "HIV treatment adherence, drug resistance, virologic failure: evolving concepts". *Infectious disorders drug targets* 11 (2): 167–74. doi:10.2174/187152611795589663. PMID 21406048.

127.   **Jump up** ^ Orsi, F; d'almeida, C (May 2010). "Soaring antiretroviral prices, TRIPS and TRIPS flexibilities: a burning issue for

antiretroviral treatment scale-up in developing countries". *Current Opinion in HIV and AIDS* **5** (3): 237–41. doi:10.1097/COH.0b013e32833860ba. PMID 20539080.

128.   **Jump up** ^ Nachega, JB; Mills, EJ; Schechter, M (January 2010). "Antiretroviral therapy adherence and retention in care in middle-income and low-income countries: current status of knowledge and research priorities". *Current Opinion in HIV and AIDS* **5** (1): 70–7. doi:10.1097/COH.0b013e328333ad61. PMID 20046150.

129.   ^ Jump up to: *a b c* Montessori, V., Press, N., Harris, M., Akagi, L., Montaner, J. S. (2004). "Adverse effects of antiretroviral therapy for HIV infection". *CMAJ* **170** (2): 229–238. PMC 315530. PMID 14734438.

130.   ^ Jump up to: *a b* Burgoyne RW, Tan DH (March 2008). "Prolongation and quality of life for HIV-infected adults treated with highly active antiretroviral therapy (HAART): a balancing act". *J. Antimicrob. Chemother.* **61** (3): 469–73. doi:10.1093/jac/dkm499. PMID 18174196.

131.   **Jump up** ^ Barbaro, G; Barbarini, G (December 2011). "Human immunodeficiency virus & cardiovascular risk". *The Indian journal of medical research* **134** (6): 898–903. doi:10.4103/0971-5916.92634. PMC 3284097. PMID 22310821.

132.   ^ Jump up to: *a b c* UNAIDS 2011 pg. 150–160

133.   ^ Jump up to: *a b* "Guidelines for the Use of Antiretroviral Agents in Pediatric HIV Infection" (PDF). *The Panel on Antiretroviral Therapy and Medical Management of HIV-Infected Children.* August 11, 2011.

134.   **Jump up** ^ *Antiretroviral therapy for HIV infection in infants and children.* World Health Organization. 2010. p. 2. ISBN 978-92-4-159980-1.

135.   **Jump up** ^ Laurence J (2006). "Hepatitis A and B virus immunization in HIV-infected persons". *AIDS Reader* **16** (1): 15–17. PMID 16433468.

136.   **Jump up** ^ Huang, L; Cattamanchi, A; Davis, JL; den Boon, S; Kovacs, J; Meshnick, S; Miller, RF; Walzer, PD; Worodria, W; Masur, H; International HIV-associated Opportunistic Pneumonias (IHOP), Study; Lung HIV, Study (June 2011). "HIV-associated Pneumocystis pneumonia". *Proceedings of the American Thoracic Society* **8** (3): 294–300. doi:10.1513/pats.201009-062WR. PMC 3132788. PMID 21653531.

137.   **Jump up** ^ "Treating opportunistic infections among HIV-infected adults and adolescents. Recommendations from CDC, the National Institutes of Health, and the HIV Medicine Association/Infectious Diseases Society of America.". Department of Health and Human Services. February 2, 2007.

138.   ^ Jump up to: *a b* Smith, [edited by] Blaine T. (2008). *Concepts in immunology and immunotherapeutics* (4th ed.). Bethesda, Md.:

American Society of Health-System Pharmacists. p. 143. ISBN 978-1-58528-127-5.

139.   **Jump up** ^ Littlewood RA, Vanable PA (September 2008). "Complementary and alternative medicine use among HIV-positive people: research synthesis and implications for HIV care". *AIDS Care* **20** (8): 1002–18. doi:10.1080/09540120701767216. PMC 2570227. PMID 18608078.

140.   **Jump up** ^ Mills E, Wu P, Ernst E (June 2005). "Complementary therapies for the treatment of HIV: in search of the evidence". *Int J STD AIDS* **16** (6): 395–403. doi:10.1258/0956462054093962. PMID 15969772.

141.   ^ Jump up to: *ᵃ ᵇ ᶜ* Irlam, JH; Visser, MM; Rollins, NN; Siegfried, N (2010-12-08). "Micronutrient supplementation in children and adults with HIV infection". In Irlam, James H. *Cochrane database of systematic reviews (Online)* (12): CD003650. doi:10.1002/14651858.CD003650.pub3. PMID 21154354.

142.   **Jump up** ^ Stone, CA; Kawai, K; Kupka, R; Fawzi, WW (November 2010). "Role of selenium in HIV infection". *Nutrition Reviews* **68** (11): 671–81. doi:10.1111/j.1753-4887.2010.00337.x. PMC 3066516. PMID 20961297.

143.   **Jump up** ^ Forrester, JE; Sztam, KA (December 2011). "Micronutrients in HIV/AIDS: is there evidence to change the WHO 2003 recommendations?". *The American journal of clinical nutrition* **94** (6): 1683S–1689S. doi:10.3945/ajcn.111.011999. PMC 3226021. PMID 22089440.

144.   ^ Jump up to: *ᵃ ᵇ* World Health Organization (May 2003). *Nutrient requirements for people living with HIV/AIDS: Report of a technical consultation*. Geneva. Archived from the original on March 25, 2009. Retrieved March 31, 2009.

145.   **Jump up** ^ Liu JP, Manheimer E, Yang M (2005). "Herbal medicines for treating HIV infection and AIDS". In Liu, Jian Ping. *Cochrane Database Syst Rev* (3): CD003937. doi:10.1002/14651858.CD003937.pub2. PMID 16034917.

146.   ^ Jump up to: *ᵃ ᵇ ᶜ* Knoll B, Lassmann B, Temesgen Z (2007). "Current status of HIV infection: a review for non-HIV-treating physicians". *Int J Dermatol* **46** (12): 1219–28. doi:10.1111/j.1365-4632.2007.03520.x. PMID 18173512.

147.   ^ Jump up to: *ᵃ ᵇ* Morgan D, Mahe C, Mayanja B, Okongo JM, Lubega R, Whitworth JA (2002). "HIV-1 infection in rural Africa: is there a difference in median time to AIDS and survival compared with that in industrialized countries?". *AIDS* **16** (4): 597–632. doi:10.1097/00002030-200203080-00011. PMID 11873003.

148.   **Jump up** ^ Zwahlen M, Egger M (2006). *Progression and mortality of untreated HIV-positive individuals living in resource-limited settings: update of literature review and evidence synthesis*

(PDF). UNAIDS Obligation HQ/05/422204. Archived from the original on April 9, 2008. Retrieved March 19, 2008.

149.   ^ Jump up to: *a b* Antiretroviral Therapy Cohort Collaboration (2008). "Life expectancy of individuals on combination antiretroviral therapy in high-income countries: a collaborative analysis of 14 cohort studies". *Lancet* **372** (9635): 293–9. doi:10.1016/S0140-6736(08)61113-7. PMC 3130543. PMID 18657708.

150.   **Jump up** ^ Schackman BR, Gebo KA, Walensky RP, Losina E, Muccio T, Sax PE, Weinstein MC, Seage GR 3rd, Moore RD, Freedberg KA. (2006). "The lifetime cost of current HIV care in the United States". *Med Care* **44** (11): 990–997. doi:10.1097/01.mlr.0000228021.89490.2a. PMID 17063130.

151.   **Jump up** ^ van Sighem, AI; Gras, LA; Reiss, P; Brinkman, K; de Wolf, F; ATHENA national observational cohort, study (2010-06-19). "Life expectancy of recently diagnosed asymptomatic HIV-infected patients approaches that of uninfected individuals". *AIDS (London, England)* **24** (10): 1527–35. doi:10.1097/QAD.0b013e32833a3946. PMID 20467289.

152.   ^ Jump up to: *a b* Cheung, MC; Pantanowitz, L; Dezube, BJ (Jun–Jul 2005). "AIDS-related malignancies: emerging challenges in the era of highly active antiretroviral therapy". *The oncologist* **10** (6): 412–26. doi:10.1634/theoncologist.10-6-412. PMID 15967835.

153.   **Jump up** ^ Tang J, Kaslow RA (2003). "The impact of host genetics on HIV infection and disease progression in the era of highly active antiretroviral therapy". *AIDS* **17** (Suppl 4): S51–S60. doi:10.1097/00002030-200317004-00006. PMID 15080180.

154.   **Jump up** ^ Lawn SD (2004). "AIDS in Africa: the impact of co-infections on the pathogenesis of HIV-1 infection". *J. Infect. Dis.* **48** (1): 1–12. doi:10.1016/j.jinf.2003.09.001. PMID 14667787.

155.   **Jump up** ^ Campbell GR, Pasquier E, Watkins J et al. (2004). "The glutamine-rich region of the HIV-1 Tat protein is involved in T-cell apoptosis". *J. Biol. Chem.* **279** (46): 48197–48204. doi:10.1074/jbc.M406195200. PMID 15331610.

156.   **Jump up** ^ Campbell GR, Watkins JD, Esquieu D, Pasquier E, Loret EP, Spector SA (2005). "The C terminus of HIV-1 Tat modulates the extent of CD178-mediated apoptosis of T cells". *J. Biol. Chem.* **280** (46): 38376–39382. doi:10.1074/jbc.M506630200. PMID 16155003.

157.   **Jump up** ^ "Tuberculosis". *Fact sheet 104*. World Health Organization. March 2012. Retrieved August 29, 2012.

158.   **Jump up** ^ World Health Organization (2011). "Global tuberculosis control 2011". ISBN 978 92 4 156438 0. Retrieved August 29, 2012.

159.   **Jump up** ^ Pennsylvania, Editors, Raphael Rubin, M.D., Professor of Pathology, David S. Strayer, M.D., Ph.D., Professor of Pathology, Department of Pathology and Cell Biology, Jefferson

Medical College of Thomas Jefferson University Philadelphia, Pennsylvania ; Founder and Consulting Editor, Emanuel Rubin, M.D., Gonzalo Aponte Distinguished Professor of Pathology, Chairman Emeritus of the Department of Pathology and Cell Biology, Jefferson Medical College of Thomas Jefferson University, Philadelphia, (2011). *Rubin's pathology : clinicopathologic foundations of medicine* (Sixth ed.). Philadelphia: Wolters Kluwer Health/Lippincott Williams & Wilkins. p. 154. ISBN 978-1-60547-968-2.

160.   **Jump up** ^ Woods, S.; Moore, D.; Weber, E.; Grant, I. (2009). "Cognitive neuropsychology of HIV-associated neurocognitive disorders". *Neuropsychology review* **19** (2): 152–168. doi:10.1007/s11065-009-9102-5. PMC 2690857. PMID 19462243. edit

161.   **Jump up** ^ Brown, T.; Qaqish, R. (2006). "Antiretroviral therapy and the prevalence of osteopenia and osteoporosis: a meta-analytic review". *AIDS (London, England)* **20** (17): 2165–2174. doi:10.1097/QAD.0b013e32801022eb. PMID 17086056. edit

162.   **Jump up** ^ Nicholas PK, Kemppainen JK, Canaval GE et al. (February 2007). "Symptom management and self-care for peripheral neuropathy in HIV/AIDS". *AIDS Care* **19** (2): 179–89. doi:10.1080/09540120600971083. PMID 17364396.

163.   **Jump up** ^ Boshoff C, Weiss R (2002). "AIDS-related malignancies". *Nature Reviews Cancer* **2** (5): 373–382. doi:10.1038/nrc797. PMID 12044013.

164.   **Jump up** ^ Yarchoan R, Tosato G, Little RF (2005). "Therapy insight: AIDS-related malignancies – the influence of antiviral therapy on pathogenesis and management". *Nat. Clin. Pract. Oncol.* **2** (8): 406–415. doi:10.1038/ncponc0253. PMID 16130937.

165.   **Jump up** ^ Post, F. .; Holt, S. . (2009). "Recent developments in HIV and the kidney". *Current opinion in infectious diseases* **22** (1): 43–48. doi:10.1097/QCO.0b013e328320ffec. PMID 19106702. edit

166.   **Jump up** ^ "AIDSinfo". *UNAIDS*. Retrieved 4 March 2013.

167.   **Jump up** ^ Cohen, MS; Hellmann, N; Levy, JA; DeCock, K; Lange, J (April 2008). "The spread, treatment, and prevention of HIV-1: evolution of a global pandemic". *The Journal of Clinical Investigation* **118** (4): 1244–54. doi:10.1172/JCI34706. PMC 2276790. PMID 18382737. Retrieved 17 September 2012.

168.   ^ Jump up to: *a b c* "UNAIDS reports a 52% reduction in new HIV infections among children and a combined 33% reduction among adults and children since 2001". *UNAIDS*. Retrieved 7 October 2013.

169.   ^ Jump up to: *a b c d* UNAIDS 2011 pg. 20–30

170.   ^ Jump up to: *a b c* UNAIDS 2011 pg. 40–50

171.   ^ Jump up to: *a b c d* Mandell, Bennett, and Dolan (2010). Chapter 117.

172.   **Jump up** ^ New HIV infections among children have been reduced by 50% or more in seven countries in sub-Saharan Africa, UN AIDS, Geneva, June 25, 2013.

173.   **Jump up** ^ Centers for Disease Control and Prevention, (CDC) (2011-06-03). "HIV surveillance—United States, 1981–2008". *MMWR. Morbidity and mortality weekly report* **60** (21): 689–93. PMID 21637182.

174.   **Jump up** ^ Health Protection Agency (2010). *HIV in the United Kingdom: 2010 Report.*

175.   **Jump up** ^ Surveillance; riques, Risk Assessment Division = Le VIH et le sida au Canada : rapport de surveillance en date du 31 décembre 2009 / Division de la surveillance et de l'évaluation des (2010). *HIV and AIDS in Canada : surveillance report to December 31, 2009.* Ottawa: Public Health Agency of Canada, Centre for Communicable Diseases and Infection Control, Surveillance and Risk Assessment Division. ISBN 978-1-100-52141-1.

176.   **Jump up** ^ "Global Report Fact Sheet". *UNAIDS.* 2010.

177.   **Jump up** ^ "COUNTRY COMPARISON :: HIV/AIDS - ADULT PREVALENCE RATE". *CIA World Factbook.* Retrieved 10 February 2014.

178.   **Jump up** ^ Gottlieb MS (2006). "Pneumocystis pneumonia— Los Angeles. 1981". *Am J Public Health* **96** (6): 980–1; discussion 982–3. doi:10.2105/AJPH.96.6.980. PMC 1470612. PMID 16714472. Archived from the original on April 22, 2009. Retrieved March 31, 2009.

179.   **Jump up** ^ Friedman-Kien AE (October 1981). "Disseminated Kaposi's sarcoma syndrome in young homosexual men". *J. Am. Acad. Dermatol.* **5** (4): 468–71. doi:10.1016/S0190-9622(81)80010-2. PMID 7287964.

180.   **Jump up** ^ Hymes KB, Cheung T, Greene JB et al. (September 1981). "Kaposi's sarcoma in homosexual men-a report of eight cases". *Lancet* **2** (8247): 598–600. doi:10.1016/S0140-6736(81)92740-9. PMID 6116083.

181.   ^ Jump up to: *a b* Basavapathruni, A; Anderson, KS (December 2007). "Reverse transcription of the HIV-1 pandemic". *The FASEB Journal* **21** (14): 3795–3808. doi:10.1096/fj.07-8697rev. PMID 17639073.

182.   **Jump up** ^ Centers for Disease Control (CDC) (1982). "Persistent, generalized lymphadenopathy among homosexual males". *MMWR Morb Mortal Wkly Rep.* **31** (19): 249–251. PMID 6808340. Retrieved August 31, 2011.

183.   **Jump up** ^ Barré-Sinoussi F, Chermann JC, Rey F et al. (1983). "Isolation of a T-lymphotropic retrovirus from a patient at risk for acquired immune deficiency syndrome (AIDS)". *Science* **220** (4599): 868–871. Bibcode:1983Sci...220..868B. doi:10.1126/science.6189183. PMID 6189183.

184.   ^ Jump up to: *a b* Centers for Disease Control (CDC) (1982). "Opportunistic infections and Kaposi's sarcoma among Haitians in the

United States". *MMWR Morb Mortal Wkly Rep.* **31** (26): 353–354; 360–361. PMID 6811853. Retrieved August 31, 2011.

185.	**Jump up ^** "Making Headway Under Hellacious Circumstances" (PDF). American Association for the Advancement of Science. July 28, 2006. Retrieved June 23, 2008.

186.	**Jump up ^** Altman LK (May 11, 1982). "New homosexual disorder worries health officials". *The New York Times.* Retrieved August 31, 2011.

187.	**Jump up ^** Kher U (July 27, 1982). "A Name for the Plague". *Time.* Archived from the original on March 7, 2008. Retrieved March 10, 2008.

188.	**Jump up ^** Centers for Disease Control (CDC) (1982). "Update on acquired immune deficiency syndrome (AIDS)—United States". *MMWR Morb Mortal Wkly Rep.* **31** (37): 507–508; 513–514. PMID 6815471.

189.	**Jump up ^** RC Gallo, PS Sarin, EP Gelmann, M Robert-Guroff, E Richardson, VS Kalyanaraman, D Mann, GD Sidhu, RE Stahl, S Zolla-Pazner, J Leibowitch, and M Popovic (1983). "Isolation of human T-cell leukemia virus in acquired immune deficiency syndrome (AIDS)". *Science* **220** (4599): 865–867. Bibcode:1983Sci...220..865G. doi:10.1126/science.6601823. PMID 6601823.

190.	**Jump up ^** Barre-Sinoussi, F.; Chermann, J.; Rey, F.; Nugeyre, M.; Chamaret, S.; Gruest, J.; Dauguet, C.; Axler-Blin, C.; Vézinet-Brun, F.; Rouzioux, C.; Rozenbaum, W.; Montagnier, L. (1983). "Isolation of a T-lymphotropic retrovirus from a patient at risk for acquired immune deficiency syndrome (AIDS)". *Science* **220** (4599): 868–871. Bibcode:1983Sci...220..868B. doi:10.1126/science.6189183. PMID 6189183. edit

191.	**Jump up ^** Aldrich, ed. by Robert; Wotherspoon, Garry (2001). *Who's who in gay and lesbian history..* London: Routledge. p. 154. ISBN 9780415229746.

192.	**Jump up ^** Gao F, Bailes E, Robertson DL et al. (February 1999). "Origin of HIV-1 in the chimpanzee Pan troglodyte's troglodytes". *Nature* **397** (6718): 436–41. Bibcode: 1999Natur.397...436G. doi:10.1038/17130. PMID 9989410.

193.	**Jump up ^** Keele, B. F., van Heuverswyn, F., Li, Y. Y., Bailes, E., Takehisa, J., Santiago, M. L., Bibollet-Ruche, F., Chen, Y., Wain, L. V., Liegois, F., Loul, S., Mpoudi Ngole, E., Bienvenue, Y., Delaporte, E., Brookfield, J. F. Y., Sharp, P. M., Shaw, G. M., Peeters, M., and Hahn, B. H. (28 July 2006). "Chimpanzee Reservoirs of Pandemic and Nonpandemic HIV-1". *Science* **313** (5786): 523–6. Bibcode:2006Sci...313..523K. doi:10.1126/science.1126531. PMC 2442710. PMID 16728595.

194.	**Jump up ^** Goodier, J., and Kazazian, H. (2008). "Retrotransposons Revisited: The Restraint and Rehabilitation of

Parasites". *Cell* **135** (1): 23–35. doi:10.1016/j.cell.2008.09.022. PMID 18854152.(subscription required)

195.	**Jump up** ^ Sharp, P. M.; Bailes, E.; Chaudhuri, R. R.; Rodenburg, C. M.; Santiago, M. O.; Hahn, B. H. (2001). "The origins of acquired immune deficiency syndrome viruses: where and when?". *Philosophical Transactions of the Royal Society B* **356** (1410): 867–76. doi:10.1098/rstb.2001.0863. PMC 1088480. PMID 11405934.

196.	**Jump up** ^ Kalish ML, Wolfe ND, Ndongmo CD, McNicholl J, Robbins KE et al. (2005). "Central African hunters exposed to simian immunodeficiency virus". *Emerg Infect Dis* **11** (12): 1928–30. doi:10.3201/eid1112.050394. PMC 3367631. PMID 16485481.

197.	^ Jump up to: *ª ᵇ* Marx PA, Alcabes PG, Drucker E (2001). "Serial human passage of simian immunodeficiency virus by unsterile injections and the emergence of epidemic human immunodeficiency virus in Africa". *Philosophical Transactions of the Royal Society B* **356** (1410): 911–20. doi:10.1098/rstb.2001.0867. PMC 1088484. PMID 11405938.

198.	**Jump up** ^ Worobey, Michael; Gemmel, Marlea; Teuwen, Dirk E.; Haselkorn, Tamara; Kunstman, Kevin; Bunce, Michael; Muyembe, Jean-Jacques; Kabongo, Jean-Marie M.; Kalengayi, Raphaël M.; Van Marck, Eric; Gilbert, M. Thomas P.; Wolinsky, Steven M. (2008). "Direct evidence of extensive diversity of HIV-1 in Kinshasa by 1960". *Nature* **455** (7213): 661–4. Bibcode:2008Natur.455..661W. doi:10.1038/nature07390. PMC 3682493. PMID 18833279. (subscription required)

199.	^ Jump up to: *ª ᵇ* Sousa, João Dinis de; Müller, Viktor; Lemey, Philippe; Vandamme, Anne-Mieke; Vandamme, Anne-Mieke (2010). "High GUD Incidence in the Early 20th Century Created a Particularly Permissive Time Window for the Origin and Initial Spread of Epidemic HIV Strains". In Martin, Darren P. *PLoS ONE* **5** (4): e9936. doi:10.1371/journal.pone.0009936. PMC 2848574. PMID 20376191.

200.	**Jump up** ^ Chitnis, Amit; Rawls, Diana; Moore, Jim (2000). "Origin of HIV Type 1 in Colonial French Equatorial Africa?". *AIDS Research and Human Retroviruses* **16** (1): 5–8. doi:10.1089/088922200309548. PMID 10628811.(subscription required)

201.	**Jump up** ^ Donald G. McNeil, Jr. (September 16, 2010). "Precursor to H.I.V. Was in Monkeys for Millennia". *New York Times*. Retrieved 2010-09-17. "Dr. Marx believes that the crucial event was the introduction into Africa of millions of inexpensive, mass-produced syringes in the 1950s. ... suspect that the growth of colonial cities is to blame. Before 1910, no Central African town had more than 10,000 people. But urban migration rose, increasing sexual contacts and leading to red-light districts."

202.	**Jump up** ^ Zhu, T., Korber, B. T., Nahmias, A. J., Hooper, E., Sharp, P. M. and Ho, D. D. (1998). "An African HIV-1 Sequence from 1959 and Implications for the Origin of the epidemic". *Nature* **391** (6667): 594–7. Bibcode:1998Natur.391..594Z. doi:10.1038/35400. PMID 9468138.

203.   **Jump up** ^ Kolata, Gina (28 October 1987). "Boy's 1969 Death Suggests AIDS Invaded U.S. Several Times". The New York Times. Retrieved 11 February 2009.

204.   ^ Jump up to: *ᵃ ᵇ* Gilbert, M. Thomas P.; Rambaut, Andrew; Wlasiuk, Gabriela; Spira, Thomas J.; Pitchenik, Arthur E.; Worobey, Michael (November 20, 2007). "The emergence of HIV/AIDS in the Americas and beyond" (PDF). *PNAS* **104** (47): 18566–18570. Bibcode:2007PNAS..10418566G. doi:10.1073/pnas.0705329104. PMC 2141817. PMID 17978186.

205.   **Jump up** ^ "The impact of AIDS on people and societies" (PDF). *2006 Report on the global AIDS epidemic*. UNAIDS. 2006. ISBN 92-9173-479-9. Retrieved June 14, 2006.

206.   **Jump up** ^ Ogden J, Nyblade L (2005). "Common at its core: HIV-related stigma across contexts" (PDF). International Center for Research on Women. Retrieved February 15, 2007.

207.   ^ Jump up to: *ᵃ ᵇ ᶜ* Herek GM, Capitanio JP (1999). "AIDS Stigma and sexual prejudice" (PDF). *American Behavioral Scientist* **42** (7): 1130–1147. doi:10.1177/0002764299042007006. Retrieved March 27, 2006.

208.   **Jump up** ^ Snyder M, Omoto AM, Crain AL (1999). "Punished for their good deeds: stigmatization for AIDS volunteers". *American Behavioral Scientist* **42** (7): 1175–1192. doi:10.1177/0002764299042007009.

209.   **Jump up** ^ Sharma, A.K. (2012). *Population and society*. New Delhi: Concept Pub. Co. p. 242. ISBN 9788180698187.

210.   **Jump up** ^ Herek, GM; Capitanio, JP; Widaman, KF (March 2002). "HIV-related stigma and knowledge in the United States: prevalence and trends, 1991–1999". *American journal of public health* **92** (3): 371–7. doi:10.2105/AJPH.92.3.371. PMC 1447082. PMID 11867313.

211.   **Jump up** ^ De Cock, KM; Jaffe, HW; Curran, JW (Jun 19, 2012). "The evolving epidemiology of HIV/AIDS". *AIDS (London, England)* **26** (10): 1205–13. doi:10.1097/QAD.0b013e328354622a. PMID 22706007.

212.   **Jump up** ^ Richard Spencer (21 August 2003). "China relaxes laws on love and marriage". *The Telegraph*. Retrieved 24 October 2013.

213.   **Jump up** ^ Bell C, Devarajan S, Gersbach H (2003). *The long-run economic costs of AIDS: theory and an application to South Africa* (PDF). World Bank Policy Research Working Paper No. 3152. Retrieved April 28, 2008.

214.   ^ Jump up to: *a b* Greener R (2002). "AIDS and macroeconomic impact". In S, Forsyth (ed.). *State of The Art: AIDS and Economics*. IAEN. pp. 49–55.

215.   **Jump up** ^ Over M (1992). *The macroeconomic impact of AIDS in Sub-Saharan Africa, Population and Human Resources Department* (PDF). The World Bank. Archived from the original on May 27, 2008. Retrieved May 3, 2008.

216.   **Jump up** ^ "AIDS Stigma". News-medical.net. Retrieved November 1, 2011.

217.   ^ Jump up to: *a b* "Thirty years after AIDS discovery, appreciation growing for Catholic approach". Catholicnewsagency.com. June 5, 2011. Retrieved November 1, 2011.

218.   ^ Jump up to: *a b* "Church HIV prayer cure claims 'cause three deaths'". BBC News. October 18, 2011. Retrieved October 18, 2011.

219.   **Jump up** ^ "Rock Hudson announces he has AIDS – History.com This Day in History – 7/25/1985". History.com. Retrieved November 1, 2011.

220.   **Jump up** ^ Coleman, Brian (June 25, 2007). "Thatcher the gay icon". *New Statesman*. Retrieved November 1, 2011.

221.   **Jump up** ^ "November 24, 1991: Giant of rock dies". *BBC On This Day* (BBC News). c. November 24, 1991. Archived from the original on October 21, 2011. Retrieved November 1, 2011.

222.   **Jump up** ^ "Freddie Mercury". Nndb.com. Retrieved November 1, 2011.

223.   **Jump up** ^ Bliss, Dominic. "Frozen In Time: Arthur Ashe". *iTENNISstore.com*. Retrieved June 25, 2012.

224.   **Jump up** ^ "Tributes to Arthur Ashe". *The Independent* (London). February 8, 1993. Retrieved July 24, 2012.

225.   **Jump up** ^ Cosgrove, Ben. "Behind the Picture: The Photo That Changed the Face of AIDS". *LIFE magazine*. Retrieved 16 August 2012.

226.   **Jump up** ^ "Aziga found guilty of first-degree murder". CTV.ca News. Retrieved 9 April 2013.

227.   **Jump up** ^ "HIV killer ruled dangerous offender". CBC News. Retrieved 9 April 2013.

228.   **Jump up** ^ "A fraudster, not a murderer". National Post. Retrieved 9 April 2013.

229.   **Jump up** ^ Duesberg, P. H. (1988). "HIV is not the cause of AIDS". *Science* **241** (4865): 514, 517. Bibcode:1988Sci...241..514D. doi:10.1126/science.3399880. PMID 3399880.Cohen, J. (1994). "The Controversy over HIV and AIDS" (PDF). *Science* **266** (5191): 1642–1649. Bibcode:1994Sci...266.1642C. doi:10.1126/science.7992043. PMID 7992043. Retrieved 2009-03-31.

230.   **Jump up** ^ Kalichman, Seth (2009). *Denying AIDS: Conspiracy Theories, Pseudoscience, and Human Tragedy*. New York:

Copernicus Books (Springer Science+Business Media). ISBN 978-0-387-79475-4.

231.   **Jump up** ^ Smith TC, Novella SP (August 2007). "HIV Denial in the Internet Era". *PLoS Med.* **4** (8): e256. doi:10.1371/journal.pmed.0040256. PMC 1949841. PMID 17713982. Retrieved 2009-11-07.

232.   **Jump up** ^ Various (January 14, 2010). "Resources and Links, HIV-AIDS Connection". National Institute of Allergy and Infectious Diseases. Retrieved 2009-02-22.

233.   **Jump up** ^ Watson J (2006). "Scientists, activists sue South Africa's AIDS 'denialists'". *Nat. Med.* **12** (1): 6. doi:10.1038/nm0106-6a. PMID 16397537.

234.   **Jump up** ^ Baleta A (2003). "S Africa's AIDS activists accuse government of murder". *Lancet* **361** (9363): 1105. doi:10.1016/S0140-6736(03)12909-1. PMID 12672319.

235.   **Jump up** ^ Cohen J (2000). "South Africa's new enemy". *Science* **288** (5474): 2168–70. doi:10.1126/science.288.5474.2168. PMID 10896606.

236.   **Jump up** ^ Boghardt, Thomas (2009). "Operation INFEKTION Soviet Bloc Intelligence and Its AIDS Disinformation Campaign". Central Intelligence Agency.

237.   **Jump up** ^ "'Virgin cure': Three women killed to 'cure' Aids". *International Herald Tribune*. February 28, 2013. Retrieved 14 September 2013.

238.   **Jump up** ^ Jenny, Carole (2010). *Child Abuse and Neglect: Diagnosis, Treatment and Evidence - Expert Consult*. Elsevier Health Sciences. p. 187. ISBN 9781437736212.

239.   **Jump up** ^ Klot, Jennifer; Monica Kathina Juma (2011). *HIV/AIDS, Gender, Human Security and Violence in Southern Africa*. Pretoria: Africa Institute of South Africa. p. 47. ISBN 0-7983-0253-4.

240.   **Jump up** ^ Blechner MJ (1997). *Hope and mortality: psychodynamic approaches to AIDS and HIV*. Hillsdale, NJ: Analytic Press. ISBN 0-88163-223-6.

241.   **Jump up** ^ Kirby DB, Laris BA, Rolleri LA (March 2007). "Sex and HIV education programs: their impact on sexual behaviors of young people throughout the world". *J Adolesc Health* **40** (3): 206–17. doi:10.1016/j.jadohealth.2006.11.143. PMID 17321420.

Bibliography

- Mandell, Gerald L.; Bennett, John E.; Dolin, Raphael, eds. (2010). *Mandell, Douglas, and Bennett's Principles and Practice of Infectious Diseases* (7th ed.). Philadelphia, PA: Churchill Livingstone/Elsevier. ISBN 978-0-443-06839-3.

Joint United Nations Programme on HIV/AIDS (UNAIDS) (2011). *Global HIV/AIDS Response, Epidemic update and health sector progress towards universal access*. Joint United Nations Programme on HIV/AIDS. The stages of HIV infection are acute infection (also known as primary infection), latency and AIDS. Acute infection lasts for several weeks and may include symptoms such as fever, swollen lymph nodes, inflammation of the throat, rash, muscle pain, malaise, and mouth and esophageal sores. The latency stage involves few or no symptoms and can last anywhere from two weeks to twenty years or more, depending on the individual. AIDS, the final stage of HIV infection, is defined by low CD4+ T cell counts (fewer than 200 per microliter), various opportunistic infections, cancers and other conditions.

Contents

[hide]

Acute infection[edit]

Main symptoms of
Acute HIV infection

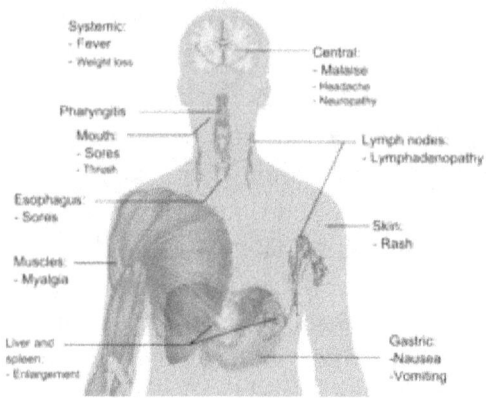

Main symptoms of acute HIV infection

Symptoms and signs of primary HIV infections[1]

	sensitivity	specificity
Fever	88%	50%
Malaise	73%	58%
Myalgia	60%	74%
Rash	58%	79%
Headache	55%	56%
Night sweats	50%	68%
Sore throat	43%	51%
Lymphadenopathy	38%	71%
Arthralgia	28%	87%
Nasal congestion	18%	60%

Acute HIV infection, primary HIV infection or acute seroconversion syndrome[2]:416) is the second stage of HIV infection. It occurs after the incubation stage, before the latency stage and the potential AIDS succeeding the latency stage.

During this period (usually 2–4 weeks post-exposure) many individuals develop an influenza or mononucleosis-like illness called acute HIV infection, the most common symptoms of which may include fever, lymphadenopathy, pharyngitis, rash, myalgia, malaise, mouth and esophageal sores, and may also include, but less commonly, headache, nausea and vomiting, enlarged liver/spleen, weight loss, thrush, and neurological symptoms. Infected individuals may experience all, some, or none of these symptoms. The duration of symptoms varies, averaging 28 days and usually lasting at least a week.[3]

Because of the nonspecific nature of these symptoms, they are often not recognized as signs of HIV infection. Even if patients go to their doctors or a hospital, they will often be misdiagnosed as having one of the more common infectious diseases with the same symptoms. As a consequence, these primary symptoms are not used to diagnose HIV infection, as they do not develop in all cases and because many are caused by other more common diseases. However, recognizing the syndrome can be important because the patient is much more infectious during this period.[1]

Latency[edit]

A strong immune defense reduces the number of viral particles in the blood stream, marking the start of secondary or chronic HIV infection. The secondary stage of HIV infection can vary between two weeks and 20 years. During this phase of infection, HIV is active within lymph nodes, which typically become persistently swollen, in response to large amounts of virus that become trapped in the follicular dendritic cells (FDC) network.[4] The surrounding tissues that are rich in CD4+ T cells may also become infected, and viral particles accumulate both in infected cells and as free virus. Individuals who are in this phase are still infectious. During this time, CD4+ CD45RO+ T cells carry most of the proviral load.[5] A small percentage of HIV-1 infected individuals retain high levels of CD4+ T-cells without antiretroviral therapy. However, most have detectable viral load and will eventually progress to AIDS without treatment. These individuals are classified as HIV controllers or long-term nonprogressors (LTNP). People who maintain CD4+ T cell counts and also have low or clinically undetectable viral load without anti-retroviral treatment are known as elite controllers or elite suppressors (ES).[6][7]

AIDS[edit]

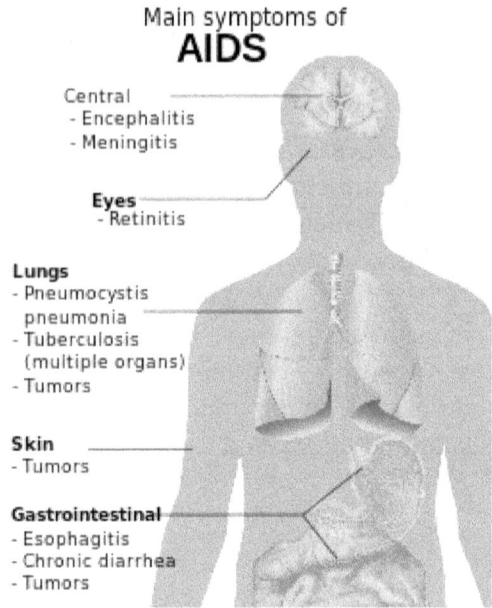

Main symptoms of AIDS.

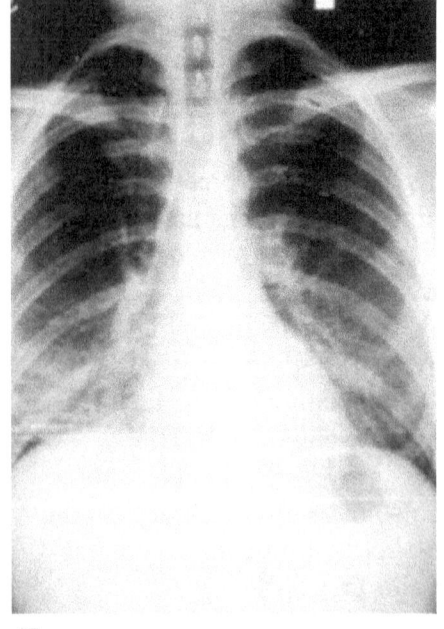

X-ray of pneumocystis pneumonia (PCP). There is increased white (opacity) in the lower lungs on both sides, characteristic of PCP.

The symptoms of AIDS are primarily the result of conditions that do not normally develop in individuals with healthy immune systems. Most of these conditions are opportunistic infections caused by bacteria, viruses, fungi and parasites that are normally controlled by the elements of the immune system that HIV damages.[8] These infections affect nearly every organ system.

People with AIDS also have an increased risk of developing various cancers such as Kaposi's sarcoma, cervical cancer and cancers of the immune system known as lymphomas. Additionally, people with AIDS often have systemic symptoms of infection like fevers, sweats (particularly at night), swollen glands, chills, weakness, and weight loss.[9][10] The specific opportunistic infections that AIDS patients develop depend in part on the prevalence of these infections in the geographic area in which the patient lives.

Pulmonary[edit]

Pneumocystis pneumonia (PCP) (originally known as *Pneumocystis carinii* pneumonia) is relatively rare in healthy, immunocompetent people, but common among HIV-infected individuals.[11] It is caused by *Pneumocystis jirovecii*.

Before the advent of effective diagnosis, treatment and routine prophylaxis in Western countries, it was a common immediate cause of death. In developing countries, it is still one of the first indications of AIDS in untested individuals, although it does not generally occur unless the CD4 count is less than 200 cells per μL of blood.[12]

Tuberculosis (TB) is unique among infections associated with HIV because it is transmissible to immunocompetent people via the respiratory route, and is not easily treatable once identified.[13] Multidrug resistance is a serious problem. Tuberculosis with HIV co-infection (TB/HIV) is a major world health problem according to the World Health Organization: in 2007, 456,000 deaths among incident TB cases were HIV-positive, a third of all TB deaths and nearly a quarter of the estimated 2 million HIV deaths in that year.[14] Even though its incidence has declined because of the use of directly observed therapy and other improved practices in Western countries, this is not the case in developing countries where HIV is most prevalent. In early-stage HIV infection (CD4 count >300 cells per μL), TB typically presents as a pulmonary disease. In advanced HIV infection, TB often presents atypically with extrapulmonary (systemic) disease a common feature. Symptoms are usually constitutional and are not localized to one particular site, often affecting bone marrow, bone, urinary and gastrointestinal tracts, liver, regional lymph nodes, and the central nervous system.[15]

Gastrointestinal[edit]

Esophagitis is an inflammation of the lining of the lower end of the esophagus (gullet or swallowing tube leading to the stomach). In HIV-infected individuals, this is normally due to fungal (candidiasis) or viral (herpes simplex-1 or cytomegalovirus) infections. In rare cases, it could be due to mycobacteria.[16]

Unexplained chronic diarrhea in HIV infection is due to many possible causes, including common bacterial (*Salmonella*, *Shigella*, *Listeria* or *Campylobacter*) and parasitic infections; and uncommon opportunistic infections such as cryptosporidiosis, microsporidiosis, *Mycobacterium avium* complex (MAC) and viruses,[17] astrovirus, adenovirus, rotavirus and cytomegalovirus, (the latter as a course of colitis).

In some cases, diarrhea may be a side effect of several drugs used to treat HIV, or it may simply accompany HIV infection, particularly during primary HIV infection. It may also be a side effect of antibiotics used to treat bacterial causes of diarrhea (common for *Clostridium difficile*). In the later stages of HIV infection, diarrhea is thought to be a reflection of changes in the way the <u>intestinal tract</u> absorbs nutrients, and may be an important component of HIV-related <u>wasting</u>.[18]

Neurological and psychiatric[<u>edit</u>]

HIV infection may lead to a variety of neuropsychiatric <u>sequelae</u>, either by infection of the now susceptible nervous system by organisms, or as a direct consequence of the illness itself.[19]

<u>Toxoplasmosis</u> is a disease caused by the single-celled <u>parasite</u> called *Toxoplasma gondii*; it usually infects the brain, causing toxoplasma <u>encephalitis</u>, but it can also infect and cause disease in the <u>eyes</u> and lungs.[20] Cryptococcal meningitis is an infection of the <u>meninx</u> (the membrane covering the brain and <u>spinal cord</u>) by the fungus *Cryptococcus neoformans*. It can cause fevers, headache, <u>fatigue</u>, <u>nausea</u>, and vomiting. Patients may also develop <u>seizures</u> and confusion; left untreated, it can be lethal.

<u>Progressive multifocal leukoencephalopathy</u> (PML) is a <u>demyelinating disease</u>, in which the gradual destruction of the <u>myelin</u> sheath covering the <u>axons</u> of nerve cells impairs the transmission of nerve impulses. It is caused by a virus called <u>JC virus</u> which occurs in 70% of the population in <u>latent</u> form, causing disease only when the immune system has been severely weakened, as is the case for AIDS patients. It progresses rapidly, usually causing death within months of diagnosis.[21]

<u>AIDS dementia complex</u> (ADC) is a metabolic <u>encephalopathy</u> induced by HIV infection and fueled by immune activation of HIV infected brain <u>macrophages</u> and <u>microglia</u>. These cells are productively infected by HIV and secrete <u>neurotoxins</u> of both host and viral origin.[22] Specific neurological impairments are manifested by cognitive, behavioral, and motor abnormalities that occur after years of HIV infection and are associated with low CD4$^+$ T cell levels and high plasma viral loads.

Prevalence is 10–20% in Western countries[23] but only 1–2% of HIV infections in India.[24][25] This difference is possibly due to the

HIV subtype in India. AIDS related mania is sometimes seen in patients with advanced HIV illness; it presents with more irritability and cognitive impairment and less euphoria than a manic episodeassociated with true bipolar disorder. Unlike the latter condition, it may have a more chronic course. This syndrome is less frequently seen with the advent of multi-drug therapy.

Tumors[edit]

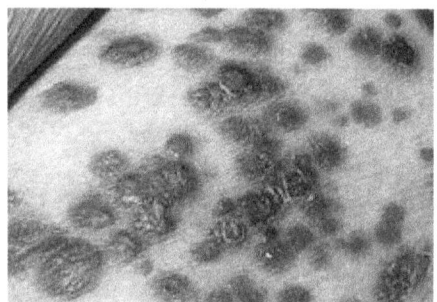

Kaposi's sarcoma

People with HIV infections have substantially increased incidence of several cancers. This is primarily due to co-infection with an oncogenic DNA virus, especially Epstein-Barr virus (EBV), Kaposi's sarcoma-associated herpesvirus (KSHV) (also known as human herpesvirus-8 [HHV-8]), and humanpapillomavirus (HPV).[26][27]

Kaposi's sarcoma (KS) is the most common tumor in HIV-infected patients. The appearance of this tumor in young homosexual men in 1981 was one of the first signals of the AIDS epidemic. Caused by a gammaherpes virus called Kaposi's sarcoma-associated herpes virus (KSHV), it often appears as purplish nodules on the skin, but can affect other organs, especially the mouth, gastrointestinal tract, and lungs. High-grade B cell lymphomas such as Burkitt's lymphoma, Burkitt's-like lymphoma, diffuse large B-cell lymphoma (DLBCL), and primary central nervous system lymphoma present more often in HIV-infected patients. These particular cancers often foreshadow a poor prognosis. Epstein-Barr virus (EBV) or KSHV cause many of these lymphomas. In HIV-infected patients, lymphoma often arises in extranodal sites such as the gastrointestinal tract.[28] When they occur in an HIV-infected patient, KS and aggressive B cell lymphomas confer a diagnosis of AIDS.

Invasive cervical cancer in HIV-infected women is also considered AIDS-defining, it is caused by human papillomavirus (HPV).[29]

In addition to the AIDS-defining tumors listed above, HIV-infected patients are at increased risk of certain other tumors, notably Hodgkin's disease, anal and rectal carcinomas, hepatocellular carcinomas, head and neck cancers, and lung cancer. Some of these are causes by viruses, such as Hodgkin's disease (EBV), anal/rectal cancers (HPV), head and neck cancers (HPV), and hepatocellular carcinoma (hepatitis B or C). Other contributing factors include exposure to carcinogens (cigarette smoke for lung cancer), or living for years with subtle immune defects.

Interestingly, the incidence of many common tumors, such as breast cancer or colon cancer, does not increase in HIV-infected patients. In areas where HAART is extensively used to treat AIDS, the incidence of many AIDS-related malignancies has decreased, but at the same time malignant cancers overall have become the most common cause of death of HIV-infected patients.[30] In recent years, an increasing proportion of these deaths have been from non-AIDS-defining cancers.

Other infections[edit]

People with AIDS often develop opportunistic infections that present with non-specific symptoms, especially low-grade fevers and weight loss. These include opportunistic infection with *Mycobacterium avium-intracellulare* and cytomegalovirus (CMV). CMV can cause colitis, as described above, and CMV retinitis can cause blindness.

Penicilliosis due to *Penicillium marneffei* is now the third most common opportunistic infection (after extrapulmonary tuberculosis and cryptococcosis) in HIV-positive individuals within the endemic area of Southeast Asia.[31]

An infection that often goes unrecognized in people with AIDS is Parvovirus B19. Its main consequence is anemia, which is difficult to distinguish from the effects of antiretroviral drugs used to treat AIDS itself.[32]

References[edit]

1. ^ Jump up to: *a b* Daar ES, Little S, Pitt J, *et al.* (2001). "Diagnosis of primary HIV-1 infection. Los Angeles County Primary HIV Infection Recruitment Network". *Annals of Internal Medicine* **134** (1): 25–9. PMID 11187417.
2. **Jump up** ^ James, William D.; Berger, Timothy G. (2006). *Andrews' Diseases of the Skin: clinical Dermatology*. Saunders Elsevier. ISBN 0-7216-2921-0.
3. **Jump up** ^ Kahn, J. O. and Walker, B. D. (1998). "Acute Human Immunodeficiency Virus type 1 infection". *N. Engl. J. Med.* **331** (1): 33–39. doi:10.1056/NEJM199807023390107. PMID 9647878.
4. **Jump up** ^ Burton GF, Keele BF, Estes JD, Thacker TC, Gartner S. (2002). "Follicular dendritic cell contributions to HIV pathogenesis". *Semin Immunol.* **14** (4): 275–284. doi:10.1016/S1044-5323(02)00060-X. PMID 12163303.
5. **Jump up** ^ Clapham PR, McKnight A. (2001). "HIV-1 receptors and cell tropism". *Br Med Bull.* **58** (4): 43–59. doi:10.1093/bmb/58.1.43. PMID 11714623.
6. **Jump up** ^ Grabar, S., Selinger-Leneman, H., Abgrall, S., Pialoux, G., Weiss, L., Costagliola, D. (2009). "Prevalence and comparative characteristics of long-term nonprogressors and HIV controller patients in the French Hospital Database on HIV". *AIDS* **23** (9): 1163–1169. doi:10.1097/QAD.0b013e32832b44c8. PMID 19444075.
7. **Jump up** ^ Blankson, J. N. (2010). "Control of HIV-1 replication in elite suppressors". *Discovery medicine* **9** (46): 261–266. PMID 20350494. edit
8. **Jump up** ^ Holmes CB, Losina E, Walensky RP, Yazdanpanah Y, Freedberg KA (2003). "Review of human immunodeficiency virus type 1-related opportunistic infections in sub-Saharan Africa". *Clin. Infect. Dis.* **36** (5): 656–662. doi:10.1086/367655. PMID 12594648.

9.   **Jump up** ^ Guss DA (1994). "The acquired immune deficiency syndrome: an overview for the emergency physician, Part 1". *J. Emerg. Med.* **12** (3): 375–384. doi:10.1016/0736-4679(94)90281-X. PMID 8040596.

10.   **Jump up** ^ Guss DA (1994). "The acquired immune deficiency syndrome: an overview for the emergency physician, Part 2". *J. Emerg. Med.* **12** (4): 491–497. doi:10.1016/0736-4679(94)90346-8. PMID 7963396.

11.   **Jump up** ^ Huang, L; Cattamanchi, A; Davis, JL; den Boon, S; Kovacs, J; Meshnick, S; Miller, RF; Walzer, PD; Worodria, W; Masur, H; International HIV-associated Opportunistic Pneumonias (IHOP), Study; Lung HIV, Study (June 2011). "HIV-associated Pneumocystis pneumonia". *Proceedings of the American Thoracic Society* **8** (3): 294–300. doi:10.1513/pats.201009-062WR. PMC 3132788. PMID 21653531.

12.   **Jump up** ^ Feldman C (2005). "Pneumonia associated with HIV infection". *Current Opinion in Infectious Diseases* **18** (2): 165–170. doi:10.1097/01.qco.0000160907.79437.5a. PMID 15735422.

13.   **Jump up** ^ Kwara A, Ramachandran G, Swaminathan S (January 2010). "Dose adjustment of the non-nucleoside reverse transcriptase inhibitors during concurrent rifampicin-containing tuberculosis therapy: one size does not fit all". *Expert Opinion on Drug Metabolism & Toxicology* **6** (1): 55–68. doi:10.1517/17425250903393752. PMC 2939445. PMID 19968575.

14.   **Jump up** ^ "Global Tuberculosis Control 2009" (PDF). Retrieved November 1, 201 1.

15.   **Jump up** ^ Decker CF, Lazarus A (August 2000). "Tuberculosis and HIV infection. How to safely treat both disorders concurrently". *Postgraduate Medicine* **108** (2): 57–60, 65–8. PMID 10951746.

16.   **Jump up** ^ Zaidi SA, Cervia JS (2002). "Diagnosis and management of infectious esophagitis associated with human immunodeficiency virus infection". *Journal of the International Association of Physicians in AIDS Care* **1** (2): 53–62. doi:10.1177/154510970200100204. PMID 12942677.

17.   **Jump up** ^ Pollok RC (2001). "Viruses causing diarrhoea in AIDS". *Novartis Foundation Symposium*. Novartis Foundation Symposia **238**: 276–83; discussion 283–8. doi:10.1002/0470846534.ch17. ISBN 978-0-470-84653-7. PMID 11444032.

18.   **Jump up** ^ Guerrant RL, Hughes JM, Lima NL, Crane J (1990). "Diarrhea in developed and developing countries: magnitude, special settings, and etiologies". *Reviews of Infectious Diseases* **12** (Suppl 1): S41–50. doi:10.1093/clinids/12.Supplement_1.S41. PMID 2406855.

19.   **Jump up** ^ Gazzard, B; Balkin, A; Hill, A (2010). "Analysis of neuropsychiatric adverse events during clinical trials of efavirenz in antiretroviral-naive patients: a systematic review". *AIDS reviews* **12** (2): 67–75. PMID 20571601. edit

20.   **Jump up** ^ Luft BJ, Chua A (August 2000). "Central Nervous System Toxoplasmosis in HIV Pathogenesis, Diagnosis, and Therapy". *Current Infectious Disease Reports* **2** (4): 358–362. doi:10.1007/s11908-000-0016-x. PMID 11095878.

21.   **Jump up** ^ Sadler M, Nelson MR (June 1997). "Progressive multifocal leukoencephalopathy in HIV". *International Journal of STD & AIDS* **8** (6): 351–7. doi:10.1258/0956462971920181. PMID 9179644.

22.   **Jump up** ^ Gray F, Adle-Biassette H, Chretien F, Lorin de la Grandmaison G, Force G, Keohane C (2001). "Neuropathology and neurodegeneration in human immunodeficiency virus infection. Pathogenesis of HIV-induced lesions of the brain, correlations with HIV-associated disorders and modifications according to treatments". *Clinical Neuropathology* **20** (4): 146–55. PMID 11495003.

23.   **Jump up** ^ Grant I, Sacktor H, McArthur J (2005). "HIV neurocognitive disorders" (PDF). In H.E. Gendelman, I. Grant, I. Everall, S. A. Lipton, and S. Swindells. (ed.). *The Neurology of AIDS* (2nd ed.). London, UK: Oxford University Press. pp. 357–373. ISBN 0-19-852610-5.

24.   **Jump up** ^ Satishchandra P, Nalini A, Gourie-Devi M et al. (January 2000). "Profile of neurologic disorders associated with HIV/AIDS from Bangalore, south India (1989–96)". *The Indian Journal of Medical Research* **111**: 14–23. PMID 10793489.

25.   **Jump up** ^ Wadia RS, Pujari SN, Kothari S et al. (March 2001). "Neurological manifestations of HIV disease". *The Journal of the Association of Physicians of India* **49**: 343–8. PMID 11291974.

26.   **Jump up** ^ Boshoff C, Weiss R (2002). "AIDS-related malignancies". *Nature Reviews Cancer* **2** (5): 373–382. doi:10.1038/nrc797. PMID 12044013.

27.   **Jump up** ^ Yarchoan R, Tosato G, Little RF (2005). "Therapy insight: AIDS-related malignancies – the influence of antiviral therapy on pathogenesis and management". *Nat. Clin. Pract. Oncol.* **2** (8): 406–415. doi:10.1038/ncponc0253. PMID 16130937.

28.   **Jump up** ^ Ho-Yen C and Chang F (June 1, 2008). "Gastrointestinal Malignancies in HIV/AIDS". *The AIDS Reader* **18** (6).

29.   **Jump up** ^ Palefsky J (2007). "Human papillomavirus infection in HIV-infected persons". *Top HIV Med* **15** (4): 130–3. PMID 17720998.

30.   **Jump up** ^ Bonnet F, Lewden C, May T et al. (2004). "Malignancy-related causes of death in human immunodeficiency

virus-infected patients in the era of highly active antiretroviral therapy". *Cancer* **101** (2): 317–324. doi:10.1002/cncr.20354. PMID 15241829.

31.   **Jump up** ^ Skoulidis, F; Morgan, MS; MacLeod, KM (August 2004). "Penicillium marneffei: a pathogen on our doorstep?". *Journal of the Royal Society of Medicine* **97** (8): 394–6. doi:10.1258/jrsm.97.8.394. PMC 1079563. PMID 15286196.

32.   **Jump up** ^ Silvero AM, Acevedo-Gadea CR, Pantanowitz L "" (June 4, 2009). "Unsuspected Parvovirus B19 Infection in a Person With AIDS". *The AIDS Reader* **19** (6).

•

AIDS is caused by the human immunodeficiency virus (HIV), which originated in non-human primates in Sub-Saharan Africa and was transferred to humans during the late 19th or early 20th century.

Two types of HIV exist: HIV-1 and HIV-2. HIV-1 is more virulent, is more easily transmitted and is the cause of the vast majority of HIV infections globally.[1] The pandemic strain of HIV-1 is closely related to a virus found in the chimpanzees of the subspecies *Pan troglodytes troglodytes*, which lives in the forests of the Central African nations of Cameroon, Equatorial Guinea, Gabon, Republic of Congo (or Congo-Brazzaville), and Central African Republic. HIV-2 is less transmittable and is largely confined to West Africa, along with its closest relative, a virus of the sooty mangabey (*Cercocebus atys atys*), an Old World monkey inhabiting southern Senegal, Guinea-Bissau, Guinea, Sierra Leone, Liberia, and western Ivory Coast.[1][2]

Contents

[hide]

Transmission from non-humans to humans[edit]

Most HIV researchers agree that HIV evolved at some point from the closely related Simian immunodeficiency virus (SIV), and that SIV or HIV (post mutation) was transferred from non-human primates to humans in the recent past (as a type of zoonosis). Research in this area is conducted using molecular phylogenetics, comparing viral genomic sequences to determine relatedness.

HIV-1 from chimpanzees and gorillas to humans[edit]

Scientists generally accept that the known strains (or groups) of HIV-1 are most closely related to the simian immunodeficiency viruses (SIVs) endemic in wild ape populations of West Central African forests. Particularly, each of the known HIV-1 strains is either closely related to the SIV that infects the chimpanzee subspecies *Pan troglodytes troglodytes* (SIVcpz) or closely related to the SIV that infects Western lowland gorillas (*Gorilla gorilla gorilla*), called SIVgor.[3][4][5][6][7][8] The pandemic HIV-1 strain (group M or Main) and a very rare strain only found in a few Cameroonian people (group N) are clearly derived from SIVcpz strains endemic in *Pan troglodytes troglodytes* chimpanzee populations living in Cameroon.[3] Another very rare HIV-1 strain (group P) is clearly derived from SIVgor strains of Cameroon.[6] Finally, the primate ancestor of HIV-1 group O, a strain infecting tens of thousands of people mostly from Cameroon but also from neighboring countries, is still uncertain, but there is evidence that it is either SIVcpz or SIVgor.[5] The pandemic HIV-1 group M is most closely related to the SIVcpz collected from the southeastern rain forests of Cameroon (modern East Province) near the Sangha River.[3] Thus, this region is presumably where the virus was first transmitted from chimpanzees to humans. However, reviews of the epidemiological evidence of early HIV-1 infection in stored blood samples, and of old cases of AIDS in Central Africa have led many scientists to believe that HIV-1 group M early human center was probably not in Cameroon, but rather farther south in the Democratic Republic of the Congo, more probably in its capital city, Kinshasa.[3][9][10][11]

Using HIV-1 sequences preserved in human biological samples along with estimates of viral mutation rates, scientists calculate that the jump from chimpanzee to human probably happened during the late 19th or early 20th century, a time of rapid urbanisation and colonisation in equatorial Africa. Exactly when the zoonosis occurred is not known. Some molecular dating studies suggest that HIV-1 group M had its most recent common ancestor (MRCA) (that is, started to spread in the human population) in the early 20th century, probably between 1915 and 1941.[12][13][14] A study published in 2008, analyzing viral sequences recovered from a recently discovered biopsy made in Kinshasa, in 1960, along with previously known sequences, suggested a common ancestor between 1873 and 1933 (with central estimates varying between 1902 and 1921).[15][16] Genetic recombination had earlier been thought to "seriously confound" such phylogenetic analysis, but later "work has suggested that recombination is not likely to systematically bias [results]", although recombination is "expected to increase variance".[15] The results of a 2008 phylogenetics study support the later work and indicate that HIV evolves "fairly reliably".[15][17]

HIV-2 from sooty mangabeys to humans[edit]

Similar research has been undertaken with SIV strains collected from several wild sooty mangabey (*Cercocebus atys atys*) (SIVsmm) communities of the West African nations of Sierra Leone, Liberia, and Ivory Coast. The resulting phylogenetic analyses show that the viruses most closely related to the two strains of HIV-2 that spread considerably in humans (HIV-2 groups A and B) are the SIVsmm found in the sooty mangabeys of the Tai forest, in western Ivory Coast.[2]

There are six additional known HIV-2 groups, each having been found in just one person. They all seem to derive from independent transmissions from sooty mangabeys to humans. Groups C and D have been found in two people from Liberia, groups E and F have been discovered in two people from Sierra Leone, and groups G and H have been detected in two people from the Ivory Coast. These HIV-2 strains are probably dead-end infections, and each of them is most closely related to SIVsmm strains from sooty mangabeys living in the same country where the human infection was found.[2][11][18]

Molecular dating studies suggest that both the epidemic groups (A and B) started to spread among humans between 1905 and 1961 (with the central estimates varying between 1932 and 1945).[19] [20]

See also this article about HIV types, groups, and subtypes.

Bushmeat practice[edit]

According to the natural transfer theory (also called 'Hunter Theory' or 'Bushmeat Theory'), the "simplest and most plausible explanation for the cross-species transmission"[7] of SIV or HIV (post mutation), the virus was transmitted from an ape or monkey to a human when a hunter or bushmeat vendor/handler was bitten or cut while hunting or butchering the animal. The resulting exposure to blood or other bodily fluids of the animal can result in SIV infection.[21] A recent serological survey showed that human infections by <u>SIV</u> are not rare in Central Africa: the percentage of people showing seroreactivity to <u>antigens</u> — evidence of current or past SIV infection — was 2.3% among the general population of <u>Cameroon</u>, 7.8% in villages where bushmeat is hunted or used, and 17.1% in the most exposed people of these villages.[22] How the SIV virus would have transformed into HIV after infection of the hunter or <u>bushmeat</u> handler from the ape/monkey is still a matter of debate, although natural selection would favor any viruses capable of adjusting so that they could infect and reproduce in the T cells of a human host.

Emergence[<u>edit</u>]

Conditions for successful zoonosis[<u>edit</u>]

<u>Zoonosis</u> (transfer of a <u>pathogen</u> from non-human animals to humans) and subsequent spread of the pathogen between humans, requires the following conditions:

1. a human population
2. a nearby population of a host animal
3. an infectious pathogen in the host animal that can spread from animal to human
4. interaction between the species to transmit enough of the pathogen to humans to establish a human foothold, which could have taken millions of individual exposures
5. ability of the pathogen to spread from human to human (perhaps acquired by <u>mutation</u>)
6. some process allowing the pathogen to disperse widely, preventing the infection from "burning out" by either killing off its human hosts or provoking immunity in a local population of humans.

Unresolved issues about HIV origins and emergence[<u>edit</u>]

It is clear that the several HIV-1 and HIV-2 strains descend from SIVcpz, SIVgor, and SIVsmm viruses,[2][5][6][7][9][18] and that bushmeat practice provides the most plausible venue for cross-species transfer to humans.[7][9][22] However, some loose ends remain unresolved.

It is not yet explained why only four HIV groups (HIV-1 groups M and O, and HIV-2 groups A and B) spread considerably in human populations, despite bushmeat practices being very widespread in Central and West Africa,[10] and the resulting human SIV infections being common.[22]

It remains also unexplained why all epidemic HIV groups emerged in humans nearly simultaneously, and only in the 20th century, despite very old human exposure to SIV (a recent phylogenetic study demonstrated that SIV is at least tens of thousands of years old).[23]

The discovery of the main HIV / SIV phylogenetic relationships permits explaining *broadly* HIV biogeography: the early centers of the HIV-1 groups were in Central Africa, where the primate reservoirs of the related SIVcpz and SIVgor viruses (chimpanzees and gorillas) exist; similarly, the HIV-2 groups had their centers in West Africa, where sooty mangabeys, which harbor the related SIVsmm virus, exist. However these relationships do not explain more detailed patterns of biogeography, such as why epidemic HIV-2 groups (A and B) only evolved in the Ivory Coast, which is only one of six countries harboring the sooty mangabey. It is also unclear why the SIVcpz endemic in the chimpanzee subspecies *Pan troglodytes schweinfurthii* (inhabiting the Democratic Republic of Congo, Central African Republic, Rwanda, Burundi, Uganda, and Tanzania) did not spawn an epidemic HIV-1 strain to humans, while the Democratic Republic of Congo was the main center of HIV-1 group M, a virus descended from SIVcpz strains of a subspecies (*Pan troglodytes troglodytes*) that does not exist in this country.

Origin and epidemic emergence[edit]

Several of the theories of HIV origin put forward (described below) attempt to explain the unresolved loose ends described in the previous section. Most of them accept the (above described) established knowledge of the HIV/SIV phylogenetic relationships, and also accept that bushmeat practice was the most likely cause of the initial transfer to humans. All of them propose that the simultaneous epidemic emergences of four HIV groups in the late 19th-early 20th century, and the lack of previous known emergences, are explained by new factor(s) that appeared in the relevant African regions in that timeframe. These new factor(s) would have acted either to increase human exposures to SIV, to help it to adapt to the human organism by mutation (thus enhancing its between-humans transmissibility), or to cause an initial burst of transmissions crossing an epidemiological threshold, and therefore increasing the odds of continued spread.

Social changes and urbanization[edit]

It was proposed by Beatrice Hahn, Paul Sharp, and colleagues that "[the epidemic emergence of HIV] most likely reflects changes in population structure and behaviour in Africa during the 20th century and perhaps medical interventions that provided the opportunity for rapid human-to-human spread of the virus".[7] After the Scramble for Africa started in the 1880s, European colonial powers established cities, towns, and other colonial stations. A largely masculine labor force was hastily recruited to work in fluvial and sea ports, railways, other infrastructures, and in plantations. This disrupted traditional tribal values, and favored sexual promiscuity. In the nascent cities women felt relatively liberated from rural tribal rules[24] and many remained unmarried or divorced during long periods,[10][25] this being very rare in African traditional societies.[26] This was accompanied by unprecedented increase in people's movements.

Michael Worobey and colleagues observed that the growth of cities had probably a role in the epidemic emergence of HIV, since the phylogenetic datations of the two older strains of HIV-1 (groups M and O), suggest that these viruses started to spread soon after the main Central African colonial cities were founded.[15]

Heart of Darkness[edit]

Amit Chitnis, Diana Rawls, and Jim Moore proposed that HIV may have emerged epidemically as a result of the harsh conditions, forced labor, displacement, and unsafe injection and vaccination practices associated with colonialism, particularly in French Equatorial Africa.[27] The workers in plantations, construction projects, and other colonial enterprises were supplied with bushmeat, this contributing to increase this activity, and then exposures to SIV. Several historical sources support the view that bushmeat hunting indeed increased, both because of the necessity to supply workers and because firearms became more widely available.[27][28][29]

The colonial authorities also gave many vaccinations against smallpox, and injections, of which many would be made without sterilising the equipment between uses (unsafe or unsterile injections). Chitnis *et al.* proposed that both these parenteral risks and the prostitution associated with forced labor camps could have caused serial transmission (or serial passage) of SIV between humans (see discussion of this in the next section).[27] In addition, they proposed that the conditions of extreme stress associated with forced labor could depress the immune system of workers, therefore prolonging the primary acute infection period of someone newly infected by SIV, thus increasing the odds of both adaptation of the virus to humans, and of further transmissions.[30]

The authors predicted that HIV-1 originated in the area of French Equatorial Africa, and in the early 20th century (when the colonial abuses and forced labor were at their peak). Later researches proved these predictions mostly correct: HIV-1 groups M and O started to spread in humans in late 19th–early 20th century.[12][13][14][15] And all groups of HIV-1 descend from either SIVcpz or SIVgor from apes living to the west of the Ubangi River, either in countries that belonged to the French Equatorial Africa federation of colonies, in Equatorial Guinea (then a Spanish colony), or in Cameroon (which was a German colony between 1884 and 1916, and then fell to Allied forces in World War I, and had most of its area administered by France, in close association with French Equatorial Africa).

This theory was later dubbed 'Heart of Darkness' by Jim Moore,[31] alluding to the book of the same title written by Joseph Conrad, the main focus of which is colonial abuses in equatorial Africa.

Unsterile injections[edit]

In several articles published since 2001, Preston Marx, Philip Alcabes, and Ernest Drucker proposed that HIV emerged because of rapid serial human-to-human transmission of SIV (after a bushmeat hunter or handler became SIV-infected) through unsafe or unsterile injections.[16][18][32][33] Although both Chitnis et al.[27] and Sharp et al.[7] also suggested that this may have been one of the major risk factors at play in HIV emergence (see above), Marx et al. enunciated the underlying mechanisms in greater detail, and wrote the first review of the injection campaigns made in colonial Africa.[18][32]

Central to Marx et al. argument is the concept of adaptation by serial passage (or serial transmission): an adventitious virus (or other pathogen) can increase its biological adaptation to a new host species if it is rapidly transmitted between hosts, while each host is still in the acute infection period. This process favors the accumulation of adaptive mutations more rapidly, therefore increasing the odds that a better adapted viral variant will appear in the host before the immune system suppresses the virus.[18] Such better adapted variant could then survive in the human host for longer than the short acute infection period, in high numbers (high viral load), which would grant it more possibilities of epidemic spread.

Marx et al. reported experiments of cross-species transfer of SIV in captive monkeys (some of which made by themselves), in which the use of serial passage helped to adapt SIV to the new monkey species after passage by three or four animals.[18]

In agreement with this model is also the fact that, while both HIV-1 and HIV-2 attain substantial viral loads in the human organism, adventitious SIV infecting humans seldom does so: people with SIV antibodies often have very low or even undetectable SIV viral load.[22] This suggests that both HIV-1 and HIV-2 are adapted to humans, and serial passage could have been the process responsible for it.

Marx et al. proposed that unsterile injections (that is, injections where the needle or syringe is reused without sterilization or cleaning between uses), which were likely very prevalent in Africa, during both the colonial period and afterwards, provided the mechanism of serial passage that permitted HIV to adapt to humans, therefore explaining why it emerged epidemically only in the 20th century.[18][32]

Massive injections of the antibiotic era[edit]

Marx et al. emphasize the massive number of injections administered in Africa after antibiotics were introduced (around 1950) as being the most likely implicated in the origin of HIV because, by these times (roughly in the period 1950 to 1970), injection intensity in Africa was maximal. They argued that a serial passage chain of 3 or 4 transmissions between humans is an unlikely event (the probability of transmission after a needle reuse is something between 0.3% and 2%, and only a few people have an acute SIV infection at any time), and so HIV emergence may have required the very high frequency of injections of the antibiotic era.[18]

The molecular dating studies place the initial spread of the epidemic HIV groups before that time (see above).[12][13][14][15][19][20] According to Marx et al., these studies could have overestimated the age of the HIV groups, because they depend on a molecular clock assumption, may not have accounted for the effects of natural selection in the viruses, and the serial passage process alone would be associated with strong natural selection.[18]

The injection campaigns against sleeping sickness[edit]

David Gisselquist proposed that the mass injection campaigns to treat trypanosomiasis (sleeping sickness) in Central Africa were responsible for the emergence of HIV-1.[34] Unlike Marx et al.,[18] Gisselquist argued that the millions of unsafe injections administered during these campaigns were sufficient to spread rare HIV infections into an epidemic, and that evolution of HIV through serial passage was not essential to the emergence of the HIV epidemic in the 20th century.[34]

This theory focuses on injection campaigns that peaked in the period 1910–40, that is, around the time the HIV-1 groups started to spread.[12][13][14][15] It also focuses on the fact that many of the injections in these campaigns were intravenous (which are more likely to transmit SIV/HIV than subcutaneous or intramuscular injections), and many of the patients received many (often more than 10) injections per year, therefore increasing the odds of SIV serial passage.[34]

Other early injection campaigns[edit]

Jacques Pépin and Annie-Claude Labbé reviewed the colonial health reports of Cameroon and French Equatorial Africa for the period 1921–59, calculating the incidences of the diseases requiring intravenous injections. They concluded that trypanosomiasis, leprosy, yaws, and syphilis were responsible for most intravenous injections. Schistosomiasis, tuberculosis, and vaccinations against smallpox represented lower parenteral risks: schistosomiasis cases were relatively few; tuberculosis patients only became numerous after mid century; and there were few smallpox vaccinations in the lifetime of each person.[35]

The authors suggested that the very high prevalence of the Hepatitis C virus in southern Cameroon and forested areas of French Equatorial Africa(around 40–50%) can be better explained by the unsterile injections used to treat yaws, because this disease was much more prevalent than syphilis, trypanosomiasis, and leprosy in these areas. They suggested that all these parenteral risks caused, not only the massive spread of Hepatitis C but also the spread of other pathogens, and the emergence of HIV-1: "the same procedures could have exponentially amplified HIV-1, from a single hunter/cook occupationally infected with SIVcpz to several thousand patients treated with arsenicals or other drugs, a threshold beyond which sexual transmission could prosper."[35] They do not suggest specifically serial passage as the mechanism of adaptation.

According to Pépin's 2011 book, *The Origins of AIDS*,[36] the virus can be traced to a central African bush hunter in 1921, with colonial medical campaigns using improperly sterilized syringe and needles playing a key role in enabling a future epidemic. Pépin concludes that AIDS spread silently in Africa for decades, fueled by urbanization and prostitution since the initial cross-species infection. Pépin also claims that the virus was brought to the Americas by a Haitian teacher returning home from Zaire in the 1960s.[37] Sex tourism and contaminated blood transfusion centers ultimately propelled AIDS to public consciousness in the 1980s and a worldwide pandemic.[36]

Genital ulcer diseases and sexual promiscuity[edit]

João Dinis de Sousa, Viktor Müller, Philippe Lemey, and Anne-Mieke Vandamme proposed that HIV became epidemic through sexual serial transmission, in nascent colonial cities, helped by a high frequency of genital ulcers, caused by genital ulcer diseases (GUD).[10] GUD are simply sexually transmitted diseases that cause genital ulcers; examples are syphilis, chancroid, lymphogranuloma venereum, and genital herpes. These diseases increase the probability of HIV transmission dramatically, from around 0.01–0.1% to 4–43% per heterosexual act, because the genital ulcers provide a portal of viral entry, and contain many activated T cells expressing the CCR5 co-receptor, the main cell targets of HIV.[10][38]

The probable time interval of cross-species transfer[edit]

Sousa *et al.* use molecular dating techniques to estimate the time when each HIV group split from its closest SIV lineage. Each HIV group necessarily crossed to humans between this time and the time when it started to spread (the time of the MRCA), because after the MRCA certainly all lineages were already in humans, and before the split with the closest simian strain, the lineage was in a simian. HIV-1 groups M and O, split from their closest SIVs around 1876 (1847–1907), 1741 (1606–1870), respectively. HIV-2 did so around 1889 (1856–1922). This information, together with the datations of the HIV groups' MRCAs (described above) mean that all HIV groups likely crossed to humans in late 19th—early 20th century.[10]

Strong GUD incidence in nascent colonial cities[edit]

The authors reviewed colonial medical articles and archived medical reports of the countries at or near the ranges of chimpanzees, gorillas and sooty mangabeys, and found that genital ulcer diseases peaked in the colonial cities during their early growth period (up to 1935). The colonial authorities recruited men to work in railways, fluvial and sea ports, and other infrastructure projects, and most of these men did not bring their wives with them. Then, the highly male-biased sex ratio favoured prostitution, which in its turn caused an explosion of GUD (especially syphilis and chancroid). After the mid-1930s, people's movements were more tightly controlled, and mass surveys and treatments (of arsenicals and other drugs) were organized, and so the GUD incidences started to decline. They declined even further after World War II, because of the heavy use of antibiotics, so that, by the late 1950s, Kinshasa (which is the probable center of HIV-1 group M) had a very low GUD incidence. Similar processes happened in the cities of Cameroon and Ivory Coast, where HIV-1 group O and HIV-2 respectively evolved.[10]

Therefore, the peak GUD incidences in cities[10] have a good temporal coincidence with the period when all main HIV groups crossed to humans and started to spread.[10][12][13][14][15][19][20] In addition, the authors gathered evidence that syphilis and the other GUDs were, like injections, absent from the densely forested areas of Central and West Africa before organized colonialism socially disrupted these areas (starting in the 1880s).[10] Thus, this theory also potentially explains why HIV emerged only after late 19th century.

Female circumcision[edit]

Uli Linke has argued that the practice of <u>female circumcision</u> is responsible for the high incidence of AIDS in Africa, since intercourse with a circumcised female is conducive to exchange of blood.[39]

Male circumcision distribution and HIV origins[edit]

Male <u>circumcision</u> may reduce the probability of HIV acquisition by men (see article <u>Circumcision and HIV</u>). Leaving aside blood <u>transfusions</u>, the highest <u>HIV-1</u> transmissibility ever measured was from GUD-suffering female prostitutes to uncircumcised men—the measured risk was 43% in a single sexual act.[38] Sousa *et al.* reasoned that the adaptation and epidemic emergence of each HIV group may have required such extreme conditions, and thus reviewed the existing <u>ethnographic</u> literature for patterns of male <u>circumcision</u> and hunting of <u>apes</u> and <u>monkeys</u> for <u>bushmeat</u>, focusing on the period 1880–1960, and on most of the 318 <u>ethnic groups</u> living in Central and West Africa.[10] They also collected censuses and other literature showing the ethnic composition of colonial cities in this period. Then, they estimated the circumcision frequencies of the Central African cities over time.

Sousa *et al.* charts reveal that male circumcision frequencies were much lower in several cities of western and central Africa in the early 20th century than they are currently. The reason is that many <u>ethnic groups</u> not performing circumcision by that time gradually adopted it, to imitate other ethnic groups and enhance the social acceptance of their boys (<u>colonialism</u> produced massive intermixing between African ethnic groups).[10][26] About 15–30% of men in <u>Kinshasa</u> and <u>Douala</u> in early 20th century should be uncircumcised, and these cities were the probable centers of HIV-1 groups M and O, respectively.[10]

The authors studied early <u>circumcision</u> frequencies in 12 cities of Central and West Africa, to test if this variable correlated with HIV emergence. This correlation was strong for HIV-2: among 6 West African cities that could have received immigrants infected with SIVsmm, the two cities from the Ivory Coast studied (Abidjan and Bouaké) had much higher frequency of uncircumcised men (60–85%) than the others, and epidemic HIV-2 groups emerged initially in this country only. This correlation was less clear for HIV-1 in Central Africa.[10]

Computer simulations of HIV emergence[edit]

Sousa *et al.* then built computer simulations to test if an 'ill-adapted SIV' (meaning a simian immunodeficiency virus already infecting a human but incapable of transmission beyond the short acute infection period) could spread in colonial cities. The simulations used parameters of sexual transmission obtained from the current HIV literature. They modelled people's 'sexual links', with different levels of sexual partner change among different categories of people (prostitutes, single women with several partners a year, married women, and men), according to data obtained from modern studies of sexual promiscuity in African cities. The simulations let the parameters (city size, proportion of people married, GUD frequency, male circumcision frequency, and transmission parameters) vary, and explored several scenarios. Each scenario was run 1,000 times, to test the probability of SIV generating long chains of sexual transmission. The authors postulated that such long chains of sexual transmission were necessary for the SIV strain to adapt better to humans, becoming a HIV capable of further epidemic emergence.

The main result was that genital ulcer frequency was by far the most decisive factor. For the GUD levels prevailing in Kinshasa, in early 20th century, long chains of SIV transmission had a high probability. For the lower GUD levels existing in the same city in the late 1950s (see above), they were much less likely. And without GUD (a situation typical of villages in forested equatorial Africa before colonialism) SIV could not spread at all. City size was not an important factor. The authors propose that these findings explain the temporal patterns of HIV emergence: no HIV emerging in tens of thousands of years of human slaughtering of apes and monkeys, several HIV groups emerging in the nascent, GUD-riddled, colonial cities, and no epidemically successful HIV group emerging in mid-20th century, when GUD was more controlled, and cities were much bigger.

Male circumcision had little to moderate effect in their simulations, but, given the geographical correlation found, the authors propose that it could have had an indirect role, either by increasing genital ulcer disease itself (it is known that syphilis, chancroid, and several other GUDs have higher incidences in uncircumcised men), or by permitting further spread of the HIV strain, after the first chains of sexual transmission permitted adaptation to the human organism.

One of the main advantages of this theory is stressed by the authors: "It [the theory] also offers a conceptual simplicity because it proposes as causal factors for SIV adaptation to humans and initial spread the very same factors that most promote the continued spread of HIV nowadays: promiscuous sex, particularly involving sex workers, GUD, and possibly lack of circumcision."[10]

Iatrogenic and other theories[edit]

Iatrogenic theories propose that medical interventions were responsible for HIV origins. By proposing factors that only appeared in Central and West Africa after the late 19th century, they seek to explain why all HIV groups also started after that.

The theories centered on the role of parenteral risks, such as unsterile injections, transfusions,[18][27][34][35] or smallpox vaccinations[27] are accepted as plausible by most scientists of the field, and were already reviewed above.

Discredited HIV/AIDS origins theories include several iatrogenic theories, such as Edward Hooper's 1999 claim that early oral polio vaccines, contaminated with a chimpanzee virus, caused the Central African outbreak.[40]

Pathogenicity of SIV in non-human primates[edit]

In most non-human primate species, natural SIV infection does not cause a fatal disease (but see below). Comparison of the gene sequence of SIV with HIV should, therefore, give us information about the factors necessary to cause disease in humans. The factors that determine the virulence of HIV as compared to most SIVs are only now being elucidated. Non-human SIVs contain a *nef* gene that down-regulates CD3, CD4, and MHC class I expression; most non-human SIVs, therefore, do not induce immunodeficiency; the HIV-1 *nef* gene, however, has lost its ability to down-regulate CD3, which results in the immune activation and apoptosis that is characteristic of chronic HIV infection.[41]

In addition, a long-term survey of chimpanzees naturally infected with SIVcpz in Gombe, Tanzania found that, contrary to the previous paradigm, chimpanzees with SIVcpz infection do experience an increased mortality, and also suffer from a Human AIDS-like illness.[42] SIV pathogenicity in wild animals could exist in other chimpanzee subspecies and other primate species as well, and stay unrecognized by lack of relevant long term studies.

History of spread[edit]

Main article: Timeline of early AIDS cases

1959: David Carr[edit]

David Carr was an apprentice printer (usually referred to, mistakenly, as a sailor; Carr had served in the Navy between 1955 and 1957) from Manchester, England who died August 31, 1959, and was for some time mistakenly reported to have died from AIDS-defining opportunistic infections. (ADOIs). Following the failure of his immune system, he succumbed to pneumonia. Doctors, baffled by what he had died from, preserved 50 of his tissue samples for inspection. In 1990, the tissues were found to be

HIV-positive. However, in 1992, a second test by AIDS researcher David Ho found that the strain of HIV present in the tissues was similar to those found in 1990 rather than an earlier strain (which would have mutated considerably over the course of 30 years). He concluded that the DNA samples provided actually came from a 1990 AIDS patient. Upon retesting David Carr's tissues, he found no sign of the virus.[43][*medical citation needed*]

1959: Congolese man[edit]

One of the earliest documented HIV-1 infections was discovered in a preserved blood sample taken in 1959 from a man from Léopoldville, Belgian Congo (now Kinshasa, Democratic Republic of the Congo).[44] However, it is unknown whether this anonymous person ever developed AIDS and died of its complications.[44]

1959: Ardouin Antonio[edit]

Considered a strong probability of HIV-infection, Ardoin Antonio was a 49-year-old shipping clerk in the garment district in Brooklyn who died of unassociated pneumocystis carinii pneumonia on June 28, 1959. The pathologist who performed his autopsy, Dr. Gordon Hennigar, insisted that Ardouin symptoms strongly suggest AIDS.

1960: Congolese woman[edit]

A second early documented HIV-1 infection was discovered in a preserved lymph node biopsy sample taken in 1960 from a woman from Leopoldville, Belgian Congo.[15]

1969: Robert Rayford[edit]

Main article: Robert Rayford

In May 1969 a 15-year-old African-American male named Robert Rayford died at the St. Louis City Hospital from Kaposi's Sarcoma. In 1987 researchers at Tulane University School of

Medicine detected "a virus closely related or identical to"[45] HIV-1 in his preserved blood and tissues. The doctors who worked on his case at the time suspected he was a prostitute, though the patient did not discuss his sexual history with them in detail.[45][46][47][48][49]

1969: Arvid Noe[edit]

Main article: Arvid Noe

In 1975 and 1976, a Norwegian sailor, with the alias name Arvid Noe, his wife, and his seven-year-old daughter died of AIDS. The sailor had first presented symptoms in 1969, eight years after he first spent time in ports along the West African coastline. A gonorrhea infection during his first African voyage shows he was sexually active at this time. Tissue samples from the sailor and his wife were tested in 1988 and found to contain HIV-1 (Group O).[50][51]

1973: Ugandan children[edit]

From 1972 to 1973, researchers drew blood from 75 children in Uganda to serve as controls for a study of Burkitt's lymphoma. In 1985, retroactive testing of the frozen blood serum indicated that antibodies to a virus related to HIV were present in 50 of the children.[52]

Spread to the western hemisphere[edit]

HIV-1 strains were once thought to have arrived in the United States from Haiti in the late 1960s or early 1970s.[53][54] HIV-1 is believed to have arrived in Haiti from central Africa, possibly through professional contacts with the Democratic Republic of the Congo.[55] The current consensus is that HIV was introduced to Haiti by an unknown individual or individuals who contracted it while working in the Democratic Republic of the Congo *circa* 1966, or from another person who worked there during that time.[54] A mini-epidemic followed, and, *circa* 1969, yet another unknown individual brought HIV from Haiti to the United States.

The vast majority of cases of AIDS outside sub-Saharan Africa can be traced back to that single patient[53] (although numerous unrelated incidents of AIDS among Haitian immigrants to the U.S. were recorded in the early 1980s, and, as evidenced by the case of Robert Rayford, isolated incidents of this infection may have been occurring as early as 1966.) The virus eventually entered male gay communities in large United States cities, where a combination of sexual promiscuity (with individuals reportedly averaging over 11 unprotected sexual partners per year[56]) and relatively high transmission rates associated with anal intercourse[57] allowed it to spread explosively enough to finally be noticed.[53]

Because of the long incubation period of HIV (up to a decade or longer) before symptoms of AIDS appear, and, because of the initially low incidence, HIV was not noticed at first. By the time the first reported cases of AIDS were found in large United States cities, the prevalence of HIV infection in some communities had passed 5%.[58] Worldwide, HIV infection has spread from urban to rural areas, and has appeared in regions such as China and India.

Canadian flight attendant theory[edit]

Main article: Gaëtan Dugas

A Canadian airline steward named Gaëtan Dugas was referred to as "Patient 0" in an early AIDS study by Dr. William Darrow of the Centers for Disease Control. Because of this, many people had considered Dugas to be responsible for bringing HIV to North America. This is not accurate, however, as HIV had spread long before Dugas began his career. This rumor may have started with Randy Shilts' 1987 book *And the Band Played On* (and the 1993 movie based on it, in which Dugas is referred to as AIDS' Patient Zero), but neither the book nor the movie states that he had been the first to bring the virus to North America. He was called "Patient Zero" because at least 40 of the 248 people known to be infected by HIV in 1983 had had sex with him, or with someone who had sexual intercourse with him.

1981: From GRID to AIDS[edit]

The AIDS epidemic officially began on June 5, 1981, when the U.S. Centers for Disease Control and Prevention in its *Morbidity and Mortality Weekly Report* newsletter reported unusual clusters of Pneumocystis pneumonia (PCP) caused by a form of *Pneumocystis carinii* (now recognized as a distinct species *Pneumocystis jirovecii*) in five homosexual men in Los Angeles.[59]

Over the next 18 months, more PCP clusters were discovered among otherwise healthy men in cities throughout the country, along with other opportunistic diseases (such as Kaposi's sarcoma[60] and persistent, generalized lymphadenopathy[61]), common in immunosuppressed patients.

In June 1982, a report of a group of cases amongst gay men in Southern California suggested that a sexually transmitted infectious agent might be the etiological agent,[62] and the syndrome was initially termed "GRID", or gay-related immune deficiency.[63]

Health authorities soon realized that nearly half of the people identified with the syndrome were not homosexual men. The same opportunistic infections were also reported among hemophiliacs,[64] heterosexual intravenous drug users, and Haitian immigrants—leading some researchers to call it the "4H" disease.[65][66]

By August 1982, the disease was being referred to by its new CDC-coined name: Acquired Immune Deficiency Syndrome (AIDS).[67]

Identification of the virus[edit]

May 1983: LAV[edit]

In May 1983, doctors from Dr. Luc Montagnier's team at the Pasteur Institute in France reported that they had isolated a new retrovirus from lymphoid ganglions that they believed was the cause of AIDS.[68] The virus was later named lymphadenopathy-associated virus (LAV) and a sample was sent to the U.S. Centers for Disease Control, which was later passed to the National Cancer Institute (NCI).[68][69]

May 1984: HTLV-III[edit]

In May 1984 a team led by Robert Gallo of the United States confirmed the discovery of the virus, but they renamed it human T lymphotropic virus type III (HTLV-III).[70]

January 1985: both found to be the same[edit]

In January 1985, a number of more-detailed reports were published concerning LAV and HTLV-III, and by March it was clear that the viruses were the same, were from the same source, and were the etiological agent of AIDS.[71][72]

May 1986: the name HIV[edit]

In May 1986, the International Committee on Taxonomy of Viruses ruled that both names should be dropped and a new name, HIV (Human Immunodeficiency Virus), be used.[73]

Nobel[edit]

Whether Gallo or Montagnier deserve more credit for the discovery of the virus that causes AIDS has been a matter of considerable controversy. Together with his colleague Françoise Barré-Sinoussi, Montagnier was awarded one half of the 2008 Nobel Prize in Physiology or Medicine for his "discovery of human immunodeficiency virus".[74] Harald zur Hausen also shared the prize for his discovery that human papilloma virus leads to cervical cancer, but Gallo was left out.[75] Gallo said that it was "a disappointment" that he was not named a co-recipient.[76] Montagnier said he was "surprised" Gallo was not recognized by the Nobel Committee: "It was important to prove that HIV was the cause of AIDS, and Gallo had a very important role in that. I'm very sorry for Robert Gallo."[75]

Classification[edit]

Since June 5, 1981, many definitions have been developed for epidemiological surveillance such as the Bangui definition and the 1994 expanded World Health Organization AIDS case definition.

Genetic studies[edit]

According to a 2008 Proceedings of the National Academy of Sciences study, a team led by Robert Shafer at Stanford University School of Medicine has discovered that the Gray Mouse Lemur has an endogenous lentivirus (the genus to which HIV belongs) in its genetic makeup. This suggests that lentiviruses have existed for at least 14 million years, much longer than the currently known existence of HIV. In addition, the time frame falls into place when Madagascar was still yet connected to what is now the African continent; the said lemurs later developed immunity to the virus strain and survived an era when the lentivirus was widespread among other mammalia. The study is being hailed as crucial, because it fills the blanks in the origin of the virus, as well as in its evolution, and may be important in the development of new antiviral drugs.[77][78]

In 2010, researchers reported that SIV had infected monkeys in Bioko for at least 32,000 years. Previous to this time, it was thought that SIV infection in monkeys had happened over the past few hundred years.[79] Scientists estimated that it would take a similar amount of time before humans adapted naturally to HIV infection in the way monkeys in Africa have adapted to SIV and not suffer any harm from the infection.[80]

Discredited hypotheses[edit]

Main article: Discredited AIDS origins theories

Other hypotheses for the origin of AIDS have been proposed. AIDS denialism argues that HIV or AIDS does not exist or that AIDS is not caused by HIV; some of its proponents believe that AIDS is caused by lifestyle, including sexuality or drug use, and not by HIV. Some conspiracy theories allege that HIV was created in a bioweapons laboratory, perhaps as an agent of genocide or an accident. These hypotheses have been rejected by scientific consensus.

See also[edit]

- Timeline of AIDS

Notes[edit]

1. ^ Jump up to: *a b* Reeves JD, Doms RW (2002). "Human immunodeficiency virus type 2". *The Journal of general virology* **83** (Pt 6): 1253–65. doi:10.1099/vir.0.18253-0 (inactive 2014-02-04). PMID 12029140.
2. ^ Jump up to: *a b c d* Santiago ML, Range F, Keele BF, Li Y, Bailes E, Bibollet-Ruche F, Fruteau C, Noë R, Peeters M, Brookfield JF, Shaw GM, Sharp PM, Hahn BH (2005). "Simian Immunodeficiency Virus Infection in Free-Ranging Sooty Mangabeys (Cercocebus atys atys) from the Tai Forest, Cote d'Ivoire: Implications for the Origin of Epidemic Human Immunodeficiency Virus Type 2". *Journal of Virology* **79** (19): 12515–27. doi:10.1128/JVI.79.19.12515-12527.2005. PMC 1211554. PMID 16160179.
3. ^ Jump up to: *a b c d* Keele BF, Van Heuverswyn F, Li Y, Bailes E, Takehisa J, Santiago ML, Bibollet-Ruche F, Chen Y, Wain LV, Liegeois F, Loul S, Ngole EM, Bienvenue Y, Delaporte E, Brookfield JF, Sharp PM, Shaw GM, Peeters M, Hahn BH (2006). "Chimpanzee Reservoirs of Pandemic and Nonpandemic HIV-1". *Science* **313** (5786): 523–6. Bibcode:2006Sci...313..523K. doi:10.1126/science.1126531. PMC 2442710. PMID 16728595.
4. **Jump up** ^ "HIV's ancestry traced to wild chimps in Cameroon". *USA Today*. 2006-05-25. Retrieved 2010-05-20.
5. ^ Jump up to: *a b c* Van Heuverswyn F, Li Y, Neel C, Bailes E, Keele BF, Liu W, Loul S, Butel C, Liegeois F, Bienvenue Y, Ngolle EM, Sharp PM, Shaw GM, Delaporte E, Hahn BH, Peeters M (2006). "Human immunodeficiency viruses: SIV infection in wild gorillas". *Nature* **444** (7116): 164. Bibcode:2006Natur.444..164V. doi:10.1038/444164a. PMID 17093443.

6.   ^ Jump up to: *a b c* Plantier JC, Leoz M, Dickerson JE, De Oliveira F, Cordonnier F, Lemée V, Damond F, Robertson DL, Simon F (2009). "A new human immunodeficiency virus derived from gorillas". *Nature Medicine* **15** (8): 871–72. doi:10.1038/nm.2016. PMID 19648927.

7.   ^ Jump up to: *a b c d e f* Sharp PM, Bailes E, Chaudhuri RR, Rodenburg CM, Santiago MO, Hahn BH (2001). "The origins of acquired immune deficiency syndrome viruses: where and when?". *Philosophical Transactions of the Royal Society B: Biological Sciences* **356** (1410): 867–76. doi:10.1098/rstb.2001.0863. PMC 1088480. PMID 11405934.

8.   **Jump up** ^ Takebe, Y; Uenishi, R; Li, X (2008). "Global Molecular Epidemiology of HIV: Understanding the Genesis of AIDS Pandemic". *HIV-1: Molecular Biology and Pathogenesis*. Advances in Pharmacology **56**. pp. 1–25. doi:10.1016/S1054-3589(07)56001-1. ISBN 9780123736017.

9.   ^ Jump up to: *a b c* Gao F, Bailes E, Robertson DL, Chen Y, Rodenburg CM, Michael SF, Cummins LB, Arthur LO, Peeters M, Shaw GM, Sharp PM, Hahn BH (1999). "Origin of HIV-1 in the chimpanzee Pan troglodyte's troglodytes". *Nature* **397** (6718): 436–441. Bibcode: 1999Natur.397...436G. Doi: 10.1038/17130. PMID 9989410.

10.   ^ Jump up to: *a b c d e f g h i j k l m n o* de Sousa JD, Müller V, Lemey P, Vandamme AM (2010). "High GUD Incidence in the Early 20th century Created a Particularly Permissive Time Window for the Origin and Initial Spread of Epidemic HIV Strains". *PLoS ONE* **5** (4): e9936. Doi: 10.1371/journal.pone.0009936. PMC 2848574. PMID 20376191.

11.   ^ Jump up to: *a b* Hooper, Edward (2000) The river : a journey to the source of HIV and AIDS Boston, MA : Little, Brown and Co ISBN 0-316-37261-7 9780316372619[*page needed*]

12.   ^ Jump up to: *a b c d e* Salami M, Strummer K, Hall WW, Duffy M, Delaporte E, Mboup S, Peeters M, Vandamme AM (2000). "Dating the common ancestor of SIVcpz and HIV-1 group M and the origin of HIV-1 subtypes by using a new method to uncover clock-like molecular evolution". *The FASEB Journal* **15** (2): 276–78. doi:10.1096/fj.00-0449fje. PMID 11156935.

13.   ^ Jump up to: *a b c d e* Korber B, Muldoon M, Theiler J, Gao F, Gupta R, Lapedes A, Hahn BH, Wolinsky S, Bhattacharya T (2000). "Timing the Ancestor of the HIV-1 Pandemic Strains". *Science* **288** (5472): 1789–96. Bibcode:2000Sci...288.1789K. doi:10.1126/science.288.5472.1789. PMID 10846155.

14.   ^ Jump up to: *a b c d e* Lemey P, Pybus OG, Rambaut A, Drummond AJ, Robertson DL, Roques P, Worobey M, Vandamme AM (2004). "The Molecular Population Genetics of HIV-1 Group O".

Genetics **167** (3): 1059–68. doi:10.1534/genetics.104.026666. PMC 1470933. PMID 15280223.

15. ^ Jump up to: *a b c d e f g h i* Worobey M, Gemmel M, Teuwen DE, Haselkorn T, Kunstman K, Bunce M, Muyembe JJ, Kabongo JM, Kalengayi RM, Van Marck E, Gilbert MT, Wolinsky SM (2008). "Direct evidence of extensive diversity of HIV-1 in Kinshasa by 1960". *Nature* **455** (7213): 661–4. Bibcode:2008Natur.455..661W. doi:10.1038/nature07390. PMC 3682493. PMID 18833279.

16. ^ Jump up to: *a b* "AIDS virus leapt the species barrier early last century: study" Breitbart, October 1, 2008. Accessed October 2, 2008.

17. **Jump up** ^ Colonial clue to the rise of HIV. BBC News. Retrieved 20-1-2009.

18. ^ Jump up to: *a b c d e f g h i j k* Marx PA, Alcabes PG, Drucker E (2001). "Serial human passage of simian immunodeficiency virus by unsterile injections and the emergence of epidemic human immunodeficiency virus in Africa". *Philos Trans R Soc Lond B Biol Sci* **356** (1410): 911–20. doi:10.1098/rstb.2001.0867. PMC 1088484. PMID 11405938.

19. ^ Jump up to: *a b c* Lemey P, Pybus OG, Wang B, Saksena NK, Salami M, Vandamme AM (2003). "Tracing the origin and history of the HIV-2 epidemic". *Proceedings of the National Academy of Sciences* **100** (11): 6588–92. Bibcode:2003PNAS..100.6588L. doi:10.1073/pnas.0936469100. PMC 164491. PMID 12743376.

20. ^ Jump up to: *a b c* Wertheim JO, Worobey M (2009). "Dating the Age of the SIV Lineages That Gave Rise to HIV-1 and HIV-2". In Drummond, Alexei J. *PLoS Computational Biology* **5** (5): e1000377. doi:10.1371/journal.pcbi.1000377. PMC 2669881. PMID 19412344.

21. **Jump up** ^ Annabel Kanabus & Sarah Allen. Updated by Bonita de Boer (2007). "The Origins of HIV & the First Cases of AIDS". AVERT (an international HIV and AIDS charity based in the UK). Retrieved 2007-02-28.

22. ^ Jump up to: *a b c d* Kalish ML, Wolfe ND, Ndongmo CB, McNicholl J, Robbins KE, Aidoo M, Fonjungo PN, Alemnji G, Zeh C, Djoko CF, Mpoudi-Ngole E, Burke DS, Folks TM (2005). "Central African hunters exposed to simian immunodeficiency virus". *Emerg Infect Dis* **11** (12): 1928–30. doi:10.3201/eid1112.050394. PMC 3367631. PMID 16485481.

23. **Jump up** ^ Worobey M, Telfer P, Souquière S, Hunter M, Coleman CA, Metzger MJ, Reed P, Makuwa M, Hearn G, Honarvar S, Roques P, Apetrei C, Kazanji M, Marx PA (2010). "Island Biogeography Reveals the Deep History of SIV". *Science* **329** (5998): 1487. Bibcode:2010Sci...329.1487W. doi:10.1126/science.1193550. PMID 20847261.

24.　　　**Jump up** ^ Egerton FC (1938) African Majesty: A Record of Refuge at the Court of the King of Bangangté in the French Cameroons. London: George Routledge & Sons.

25.　　　**Jump up** ^ Gondola, Charles Didier (1996). *Villes miroirs: migrations et identités urbaines à Kinshasa et Brazzaville, 1930–1970* (in French). Paris: L'Harmattan. ISBN 978-2-7384-4868-2.^[page needed]

26.　　　^ Jump up to: ^{*a b*} Friedrichs A (Herzogs zu Mecklenbourg), editor (1924) Wissenschaftliche Ergebnisse der Deutschen Zentral-Afrika Expedition 1907–1908. Leipzig: Klinkhardt & Biermann.

27.　　　^ Jump up to: ^{*a b c d e f*} Chitnis A, Rawls D, Moore J (2000). "Origin of HIV Type 1 in Colonial French Equatorial Africa?". *AIDS Research and Human Retroviruses* 16 (1): 5–8. doi:10.1089/088922200309548. PMID 10628811.

28.　　　**Jump up** ^ Merfield FG (1957) Gorillas were my Neighbours. London: The Company Book Club.

29.　　　**Jump up** ^ Coquery-Vidrovitch C (1998). "The Upper-Sangha in the Time of the Concession Companies". *Yale F & ES Bulletin* **102**: 72–84.

30.　　　**Jump up** ^ Moore J (2001) About this paper and comments on 'The River' url=http://weber.ucsd.edu/~jmoore/publications/HIVorigin.html

31.　　　**Jump up** ^ Moore J (2004). "The Puzzling Origins of AIDS". *American Scientist* **92**: 540–47. doi:10.1511/2004.6.540.

32.　　　^ Jump up to: ^{*a b c*} Drucker E, Alcabes PG, Marx PA (2001). "The injection century: massive unsterile injections and the emergence of human pathogens". *Lancet* **358** (9297): 1989–92. doi:10.1016/S0140-6736(01)06967-7. PMID 11747942.

33.　　　**Jump up** ^ Donald G. McNeil, Jr. (September 16, 2010). "Precursor to H.I.V. Was in Monkeys for Millennia". *New York Times*. Retrieved 2010-09-17. "Dr. Marx believes that the crucial event was the introduction into Africa of millions of inexpensive, mass-produced syringes in the 1950s. ... suspect that the growth of colonial cities is to blame. Before 1910, no Central African town had more than 10,000 people. But urban migration rose, increasing sexual contacts and leading to red-light districts."

34.　　　^ Jump up to: ^{*a b c d*} Gisselquist D (2003). "Emergence of the HIV type 1 epidemic in the twentieth century: comparing hypotheses to evidence". *AIDS Res Hum Retroviruses* **19** (12): 1071–78. doi:10.1089/088922203771881158. PMID 14709242.

35.　　　^ Jump up to: ^{*a b c*} Pépin J, Labbé AC (2008). "Noble goals, unforeseen consequences: control of tropical diseases in colonial Central Africa and the iatrogenic transmission of blood-borne viruses". *Trop Med Int Health* **13** (6): 744–53. doi:10.1111/j.1365-3156.2008.02060.x. PMID 18397182.

36.　　　^ Jump up to: ^{*a b*} Pépin, Jacques (2011). *The Origins of AIDS*. Cambridge University Press. ISBN 978-0-521-18637-7.

37.   **Jump up** ^ Jacques Pépin (2011). *The Origins of AIDS*. Cambridge University Press. p. 311. ISBN 978-0-521-18637-7.

38.   ^ Jump up to: *a b* Cameron DW, Simonsen JN, D'Costa LJ, Ronald AR, Maitha GM, Gakinya MN, Cheang M, Ndinya-Achola JO, Piot P, Brunham RC (1989). "Female to male transmission of human immunodeficiency virus type 1: risk factors for seroconversion in men". *Lancet* **334** (8660): 403–407. doi:10.1016/S0140-6736(89)90589-8. PMID 2569597.

39.   **Jump up** ^ Linke, Uli (January 1986). "AIDS in Africa". *Science* **231** (4735): 203. Bibcode:1986Sci...231..203L. doi:10.1126/science.231.4735.203-b.

40.   **Jump up** ^ Sarah Ramsay 28 April 2001 "Cold water downstream from The River" *The Lancet* **357** (9265) p.1343 doi:10.1016/S0140-6736(00)04536-0

41.   **Jump up** ^ Schindler M, Münch J, Kutsch O, Li H, Santiago ML, Bibollet-Ruche F, Müller-Trutwin MC, Novembre FJ, Peeters M, Courgnaud V, Bailes E, Roques P, Sodora DL, Silvestri G, Sharp PM, Hahn BH, Kirchhoff F (2006). "Nef-mediated suppression of T cell activation was lost in a lentiviral lineage that gave rise to HIV-1". *Cell* **125** (6): 1055–67. doi:10.1016/j.cell.2006.04.033. PMID 16777597.

42.   **Jump up** ^ Keele BF, Jones JH, Terio KA, Estes JD, Rudicell RS, Wilson ML, Li Y, Learn GH, Beasley TM, Schumacher-Stankey J, Wroblewski E, Mosser A, Raphael J, Kamenya S, Lonsdorf EV, Travis DA, Mlengeya T, Kinsel MJ, Else JG, Silvestri G, Goodall J, Sharp PM, Shaw GM, Pusey AE, Hahn BH (2009). "Increased mortality and AIDS-like immunopathology in wild chimpanzees infected with SIVcpz". *Nature* **460** (7254): 515–19. Bibcode:2009Natur.460..515K. doi:10.1038/nature08200. PMC 2872475. PMID 19626114.

43.   **Jump up** ^ Steve Connor (March 24, 1995). "How scientists discovered false evidence on the world's "first AIDS victim"". *The Independent*. Retrieved February 13, 2012.

44.   ^ Jump up to: *a b* Zhu T, Korber BT, Nahmias AJ, Hooper E, Sharp PM, Ho DD (1998). "An African HIV-1 Sequence from 1959 and Implications for the Origin of the Epidemic". *Nature* **391** (6667): 594–7. Bibcode:1998Natur.391..594Z. doi:10.1038/35400. PMID 9468138.

45.   ^ Jump up to: *a b* Garry RF, Witte MH, Gottlieb AA, Elvin-Lewis M, Gottlieb MS, Witte CL, Alexander SS, Cole WR, Drake WL (October 1988). "Documentation of an AIDS virus infection in the United States in 1968". *JAMA* **260** (14): 2085–7. doi:10.1001/jama.260.14.2085. PMID 3418874.

46.   **Jump up** ^ Haislip AM, Witte MH, Sullivan KA, Wolfe M, Gottlieb AA, Gottlieb MS, Cole WR, Witte CL, Garry RF. "The Earliest Known AIDS Patient in the United States was Infected with an HIV-1 Strain Closely Related to IIIB/LAI". *XIth International*

Congress of Virology, Sydney Convention Center, Australia, 9–13 August 1999. Archived from the original on 2007-04-15.

47.   **Jump up** ^ http://hivinsite.ucsf.edu/InSite?page=kb-01-03

48.   **Jump up** ^ http://ww2.aegis.org/news/ct/1987/CT871003.html

49.   **Jump up** ^ Kolata, Gina (1987-10-28). "Boy's 1969 death suggests AIDS invaded U.S. Several times". *The New York Times.*

50.   **Jump up** ^ Frøland SS, Jenum P, Lindboe CF, Wefring KW, Linnestad PJ, Böhmer T (June 1988). "HIV-1 infection in Norwegian family before 1970". *Lancet* **1** (8598): 1344–5. doi:10.1016/S0140-6736(88)92164-2. PMID 2897596.

51.   **Jump up** ^ Hooper E (1997). "Sailors and star-bursts, and the arrival of HIV". *BMJ* **315** (7123): 1689–91. doi:10.1136/bmj.315.7123.1689. PMC 2128008. PMID 9448543.

52.   **Jump up** ^ Saxinger WC, Levine PH, Dean AG, de Thé G, Lange-Wantzin G, Moghissi J, Laurent F, Hoh M, Sarngadharan MG, Gallo RC (March 1985). "Evidence for exposure to HTLV-III in Uganda before 1973". *Science* **227** (4690): 1036–1038. doi:10.1126/science.2983417. PMID 2983417.

53.   ^ Jump up to: *a b c* Gilbert MT, Rambaut A, Wlasiuk G, Spira TJ, Pitchenik AE, Worobey M (2007). "The emergence of HIV/AIDS in the Americas and beyond". *Proc Natl Acad Sci USA* **104** (47): 18566–70. Bibcode:2007PNAS..10418566G. doi:10.1073/pnas.0705329104. PMC 2141817. PMID 17978186.

54.   ^ Jump up to: *a b* "Key HIV strain 'came from Haiti'". *BBC News.* 2007-10-30. Retrieved 2010-05-20.

55.   **Jump up** ^ Study Says AIDS in U.S. Earlier than Thought

56.   **Jump up** ^ Morris M, Dean L (1994). "Effect of sexual behavior change on long-term human immunodeficiency virus prevalence among homosexual men". *American Journal of Epidemiology* **140** (3): 217–232. PMID 8030625.

57.   **Jump up** ^ Jin F, Jansson J, Law M, Prestage GP, Zablotska I, Imrie JC, Kippax SC, Kaldor JM, Grulich AE, Wilson DP (March 2010). "Per-contact probability of HIV transmission in homosexual men in Sydney in the era of HAART". *AIDS* **24** (6): 907–913. doi:10.1097/QAD.0b013e3283372d90. PMC 2852627. PMID 20139750. Retrieved 2010-04-11.

58.   **Jump up** ^ Jaffe HW, Darrow WW, Echenberg DF, O'Malley PM, Getchell JP, Kalyanaraman VS, Byers RH, Drennan DP, Braff EH, Curran JW (1985). "The acquired immunodeficiency syndrome in a cohort of homosexual men. A six-year follow-up study". *Annals of Internal Medicine* **103** (2): 210–4. doi:10.7326/0003-4819-103-2-210. PMID 2990275.

59.   **Jump up** ^ "Pneumocystis pneumonia—Los Angeles". *MMWR Morb. Mortal. Wkly. Rep.* **30** (21): 250–2. June 1981. PMID 6265753.

60.   **Jump up** ^ "Update on Kaposi's sarcoma and opportunistic infections in previously healthy persons—United States". *MMWR Morb. Mortal. Wkly. Rep.* **31** (22): 294, 300–1. June 1982. PMID 6810086.

61.   **Jump up** ^ "Persistent, generalized lymphadenopathy among homosexual males". *MMWR Morb. Mortal. Wkly. Rep.* **31** (19): 249–51. May 1982. PMID 6808340.

62.   **Jump up** ^ "A cluster of Kaposi's sarcoma and *Pneumocystis carinii* pneumonia among homosexual male residents of Los Angeles and Orange Counties, California". *MMWR Morb. Mortal. Wkly. Rep.* **31** (23): 305–7. June 1982. PMID 6811844.

63.   **Jump up** ^ Clue Found on Homosexuals' Precancer Syndrome — The New York Times, June 18, 1982

64.   **Jump up** ^ "*Pneumocystis carinii* pneumonia among persons with hemophilia A". *MMWR Morb. Mortal. Wkly. Rep.* **31** (27): 365–7. July 1982. PMID 6815443.

65.   **Jump up** ^ "Opportunistic infections and Kaposi's sarcoma among Haitians in the United States". *MMWR Morb. Mortal. Wkly. Rep.* **31** (26): 353–4, 360–1. July 1982. PMID 6811853.

66.   **Jump up** ^ Cohen J (2006). "HIV/AIDS: Latin America & Caribbean. HAITI: making headway under hellacious circumstances". *Science* **313** (5786): 470–3. doi:10.1126/science.313.5786.470b. PMID 16873641.

67.   **Jump up** ^ Marx JL (August 1982). "New disease baffles medical community". *Science* **217** (4560): 618–21. Bibcode:1982Sci...217..618M. doi:10.1126/science.7089584. PMID 7089584.

68.   ^ Jump up to: *a b* Barré-Sinoussi F, Chermann JC, Rey F, Nugeyre MT, Chamaret S, Gruest J, Dauguet C, Axler-Blin C, Vézinet-Brun F, Rouzioux C, Rozenbaum W, Montagnier L (1983). "Isolation of a T-lymphotropic retrovirus from a patient at risk for acquired immune deficiency syndrome (AIDS)". *Science* **220** (4599): 868–71. Bibcode:1983Sci...220..868B. doi:10.1126/science.6189183. PMID 6189183.

69.   **Jump up** ^ Kingman, Sharon; Connor, Steve (1989). *The search for the virus*. Harmondsworth [Eng.]: Penguin. ISBN 0-14-011397-5.

70.   **Jump up** ^ Popovic M, Sarngadharan MG, Read E, Gallo RC (1984). "Detection, isolation, and continuous production of cytopathic retroviruses (HTLV-III) from patients with AIDS and pre-AIDS". *Science* **224** (4648): 497–500. Bibcode:1984Sci...224..497P. doi:10.1126/science.6200935. PMID 6200935.

71.   **Jump up** ^ Marx JL (March 1985). "A virus by any other name . .". *Science* **227** (4693): 1449–51. Bibcode:1985Sci...227.1449M. doi:10.1126/science.2983427. PMID 2983427.

72.   **Jump up ^** Chang SY, Bowman BH, Weiss JB, Garcia RE, White TJ (June 1993). "The origin of HIV-1 isolate HTLV-IIIB". *Nature* **363** (6428): 466–9. doi:10.1038/363466a0. PMID 8502298.

73.   **Jump up ^** Coffin J, Haase A, Levy JA, Montagnier L, Oroszlan S, Teich N, Temin H, Toyoshima K, Varmus H, Vogt P (1986). "What to call the AIDS virus?". *Nature* **321** (6065): 10. Bibcode:1986Natur.321...10.. doi:10.1038/321010a0. PMID 3010128.

74.   **Jump up ^** "The Nobel Prize in Physiology or Medicine 2008". Nobel Foundation. Retrieved October 28, 2009.

75.   ^ Jump up to: *a b* Cohen J, Enserink M (10 October 2008). "Nobel Prize in Physiology or Medicine: HIV, HPV researchers honored, but one scientist is left out". *Science* **322** (5899): 149–175. doi:10.1126/science.322.5899.174. PMID 18845715.

76.   **Jump up ^** Altman, Lawrence (2008-10-06). "Three Europeans Win the 2008 Nobel for Medicine". New York Times. Retrieved 2008-10-06.

77.   **Jump up ^** Gifford RJ, Katzourakis A, Tristem M, Pybus OG, Winters M, Shafer RW (December 2008). "A transitional endogenous lentivirus from the genome of a basal primate and implications for lentivirus evolution". *Proc. Natl. Acad. Sci. U.S.A.* **105** (51): 20362–7. Bibcode:2008PNAS..10520362G. doi:10.1073/pnas.0807873105. PMC 2603253. PMID 19075221.

78.   **Jump up ^** Beaumont, Peter (2008-12-18). "Primate offers missing link to ancestor of the Aids virus". *The Guardian* (London). Retrieved 2008-12-19.

79.   **Jump up ^** McNeil Jr, Donald (17 September 2010). "Precursor to H.I.V. Was in Monkeys for Millenniums". *The New York Times*. Retrieved 17 September 2010.

80.   **Jump up ^** "HIV precursor in monkeys ancient: study". CBC News. 17 September 2010. Retrieved 17 September 2010.

HIV/AIDS denialism is the belief, contradicted by conclusive medical and scientific evidence,[1][2] that human immunodeficiency virus (HIV) does not cause acquired immune deficiency syndrome (AIDS).[3] Some denialists reject the existence of HIV, while others accept that HIV exists but say that it is a harmless passenger virus and not the cause of AIDS. Insofar as denialists acknowledge AIDS as a real disease, they attribute it to some combination of sexual behavior, recreational drugs, malnutrition, poor sanitation, haemophilia, or the effects of the drugs used to treat HIV infection.[4][5]

The scientific consensus is that the evidence showing HIV to be the cause of AIDS is conclusive[1][2] and that AIDS-denialist claims are pseudoscience based on conspiracy theories,[6] faulty reasoning, cherry picking, and misrepresentation of mainly outdated scientific data.[1][2][7] With the rejection of these arguments by the scientific community, AIDS-denialist material is now targeted at less scientifically sophisticated audiences and spread mainly through the Internet.[8][9]

Despite its lack of scientific acceptance, HIV/AIDS denialism has had a significant political impact, especially in South Africa under the presidency of Thabo Mbeki. Scientists and physicians have raised alarm at the human cost of HIV/AIDS denialism, which discourages HIV-positive people from using proven treatments.[2][6][8][10][11][12] Public health researchers have attributed 330,000 to 340,000 AIDS deaths, along with 171,000 other HIV infections and 35,000 infant HIV infections, to the South African government's former embrace of HIV/AIDS denialism.[13][14]

Contents

History[edit]

In 1983, a group of scientists and doctors at the Pasteur Institute in France, led by Luc Montagnier, discovered a new virus in a patient with signs and symptoms that often preceded AIDS.[15] They named the virus *lymphadenopathy-associated virus*, or LAV, and sent samples to Robert Gallo's team in the United States. Their findings were peer reviewed and slated for publication in *Science*.

At a 23 April 1984 press conference in Washington, D.C., Margaret Heckler, Secretary of Health and Human Services, announced that Gallo and his co-workers had discovered a virus that is the "probable" cause of AIDS. This virus was initially named HTLV-III.[16] That same year, Casper Schmidt responded to Gallo's papers with "The Group-Fantasy Origins of AIDS", *Journal of Psychohistory*.[17] Schmidt posited that AIDS was not an actual disease, but rather an example of "epidemic hysteria" in which groups of people are subconsciously acting out social conflicts. Schmidt compared AIDS to documented cases of epidemic hysteria in the past which were mistakenly thought to be infectious. (Schmidt himself would later die of AIDS in 1994.)[18][19]

In 1986, the viruses discovered by Montagnier and Gallo, found to be genetically indistinguishable, were renamed HIV.[20]

In 1987, Peter Duesberg questioned the link between HIV and AIDS in the journal *Cancer Research*.[21] Duesberg's publication coincided with the start of major public health campaigns and the development of zidovudine (AZT) as a treatment for HIV/AIDS.

In 1988, a panel of the Institute of Medicine of the U.S. National Academy of Sciences found that "the evidence that HIV causes

AIDS is scientifically conclusive."[1] That same year, *Science* published Blattner, Gallo, and Temin's *HIV causes AIDS*,[22] and Peter Duesberg's *HIV is not the cause of AIDS*.[23] Also that same year, The Perth Group, a group of denialists based in Perth, Western Australia led by Eleni Papadopulos-Eleopulos, published in the non-peer-reviewed journal *Medical Hypotheses* their first article questioning aspects of HIV/AIDS research,[24] arguing that there was "no compelling reason for preferring the viral hypothesis of AIDS to one based on the activity of oxidising agents."

In 1989, Duesberg exercised his right, as a member of the National Academy of Sciences, to bypass the peer review process and publish his arguments in *Proceedings of the National Academy of Sciences of the United States of America* (*PNAS*) unreviewed. The editor of *PNAS* initially resisted, but ultimately allowed Duesberg to publish, saying: "If you wish to make these unsupported, vague, and prejudicial statements in print, so be it. But I cannot see how this would be convincing to any scientifically trained reader."[25]

In 1990, Robert Root-Bernstein published his first peer-reviewed article detailing his objections to the mainstream view of AIDS and HIV.[26] In it, he questioned both the mainstream view and the "dissident" view as potentially inaccurate.

In 1991, The Group for the Scientific Reappraisal of the HIV-AIDS Hypothesis, comprising twelve scientists, doctors, and activists, submitted a short letter to various journals, but the letter was rejected.

In 1993, *Nature* published an editorial arguing that Duesberg had forfeited his right of reply by engaging in disingenuous rhetorical techniques and ignoring any evidence that conflicted with his claims.[27] That same year, Papadopulos-Eleopulos et al. of the Perth Group, alleged in the journal *Nature Biotechnology* (then edited by fellow denialist Harvey Bialy) that the Western blot test for HIV was not standardized, non-reproducible, and of unknown specificity due to a claimed lack of a "gold standard".[28][29]

On 28 October 1994, <u>Robert Willner</u>, a physician whose medical license had been revoked for, among other things, treating an AIDS patient with <u>ozone therapy</u>, publicly jabbed his finger with blood he said was from an HIV-infected patient.[6] Willner died in 1995 of a heart attack.[30]

In 1995, a letter, similar to the one submitted by The Group for the Scientific Reappraisal of the HIV-AIDS Hypothesis in 1991, was published in *Science*.[31] That same year, Continuum, a denialist group, placed an advertisement in the British gay and lesbian magazine *The Pink Paper* offering a £1,000 reward to "the first person finding one scientific paper establishing actual isolation of HIV", according to a set of seven steps they claimed to have been drawn up by the Pasteur Institute in 1973.[32] The challenge was later dismissed by various scientists, including Duesberg, asserting that HIV undoubtedly exists.[32]

In 1996, the *British Medical Journal* published *Response: arguments contradict the "foreign protein-zidovudine" hypothesis*[33] as a response to a petition by Peter Duesberg: "In 1991 Duesberg challenged researchers… We and Darby et al. have provided that evidence". The paper argued that Duesberg was wrong regarding the cause of AIDS in haemophiliacs. In 1997, The Perth Group questioned the existence of HIV, and speculated that the production of antibodies recognizing HIV proteins can be caused by allogenic stimuli and <u>autoimmune disorders</u>.[34][35] They continued to repeat this speculation through at least 2006.[36]

In 2006, <u>Celia Farber</u>, a journalist and prominent HIV/AIDS denialist, published an essay in the March issue of *Harper's Magazine* entitled "Out of Control: AIDS and the Corruption of Medical Science", in which she summarized a number of arguments for HIV/AIDS denialism and alleged incompetence, <u>conspiracy</u>, and fraud on the part of the medical community.[37] Scientists and AIDS activists extensively criticized the article as inaccurate, misleading, and poorly fact-checked.[38][39]

In 2007, members of the Perth Group testified at an appeals

hearing for <u>Andre Chad Parenzee</u>, asserting that HIV could not be transmitted by heterosexual sex. The judge concluded, "I reject the evidence of Ms Papadopulos-Eleopulos and Dr Turner. I conclude... that they are not qualified to give expert opinions."[40]

In U.S. courts[edit]

In 1998, HIV/AIDS denialism and parental rights clashed with the medical establishment in court when Maine resident Valerie Emerson fought for the right to refuse to give AZT to her four-year-old son, Nikolas Emerson, after she witnessed the death of her daughter Tia, who died at the age of three in 1996. Her right to stop treatment was upheld by the court in light of "her unique experience."[41] Nikolas Emerson died eight years later. The family refused to reveal whether the death was AIDS related.[42]

In South Africa[edit]

In 2000, South Africa's President <u>Thabo Mbeki</u> invited several HIV/AIDS denialists to join his Presidential AIDS Advisory Panel.[43] A response named the <u>Durban Declaration</u> was issued affirming the <u>scientific consensus</u> that HIV causes AIDS:

> "The declaration has been signed by over 5,000 people, including Nobel prizewinners, directors of leading research institutions, scientific academies and medical societies, notably the US National Academy of Sciences, the US Institute of Medicine, Max Planck institutes, the European Molecular Biology Organization, the Pasteur Institute in Paris, the Royal Society of London, the AIDS Society of India and the National Institute of Virology in South Africa. In addition, thousands of individual scientists and doctors have signed, including many from the countries bearing the greatest burden of the epidemic. Signatories are of MD, PhD level or equivalent, although scientists working for commercial companies were asked not to sign."[12]

In 2008, University of Cape Town researcher Nicoli Nattrass, and later that year a group of Harvard scientists led by Zimbabwean physician Pride Chigwedere each independently estimated that Thabo Mbeki's denialist policies led to the early deaths of more than 330,000 South Africans.[13][14] Barbara Hogan, the health minister appointed by Mbeki's successor, voiced shame over the studies' findings and stated: "The era of denialism is over completely in South Africa."[44]

HIV/AIDS denialists' claims and scientific evidence[edit]

See also: Duesberg hypothesis

Although members of the HIV/AIDS denialist community are united by their disagreement with the concept that HIV is the cause of AIDS, the specific positions taken by various groups differ. Denialists claim many incompatible things: HIV does not exist; HIV has not been adequately isolated,[45] HIV does not fulfill Koch's postulates,[46] HIV testing is inaccurate,[28] and that antibodies to HIV neutralize the virus and render it harmless.[47] Suggested alternative causes of AIDS include recreational drugs, malnutrition, and the very antiretroviral drugs used to treat the syndrome.[48]

Such claims have been examined extensively in the peer-reviewed medical and scientific literature; a scientific consensus has arisen that denialist claims have been convincingly disproved, and that HIV does indeed cause AIDS.[2][49] In the cases cited by Duesberg where HIV "cannot be isolated", PCR or other techniques demonstrate the presence of the virus,[50] and denialist claims of HIV test inaccuracy result from an incorrect or outdated understanding of how HIV antibody testing is performed and interpreted.[51][52] Regarding Koch's postulates, *New Scientist* reported: "It is debatable how appropriate it is to focus on a set of principles devised for bacterial infections in a century when viruses had not yet been discovered. HIV does, however, meet

Koch's postulates as long as they are not applied in a ridiculously stringent way". The author then demonstrated how each postulate has been met – the suspected cause is strongly associated with the disease, the suspected pathogen can be both isolated and spread outside the host, and when the suspected pathogen is transmitted to a new and uninfected host, that host develops the disease.[2][53] The latter was proven in a number of tragic accidents, including an instance when multiple scientific technicians with no other known risk factors were exposed to concentrated HIV virus in a laboratory accident, and transmission by a dentist to patients, the majority of whom had no other known risk factor or source of exposure except the same dentist in common.[2]

Early denialist arguments held that the HIV/AIDS paradigm was flawed because it had not led to effective treatments. However, the introduction of highly active antiretroviral therapy in the mid-1990s and dramatic improvements in survival of HIV/AIDS patients reversed this argument, as these treatments were based directly on anti-viral activity and the HIV/AIDS paradigm.[54] The development of effective anti-AIDS therapies based on targeting of the HIV virus has been a major factor in convincing some denialist scientists to accept the causative role of HIV in AIDS.[55]

In a 2010 article on conspiracy theories in science, Ted Goertzel lists HIV/AIDS denialism as an example where scientific findings are being disputed on irrational grounds. He describes proponents as relying on rhetoric, appeal to fairness, and the right to a dissenting opinion rather than on evidence. They frequently invoke the meme of a "courageous independent scientist resisting orthodoxy", invoking the name of persecuted physicist and astronomer Galileo Galilei.[56] Regarding this comparison, Goertzel states:

...being a dissenter from orthodoxy is not difficult; the hard part is actually having a better theory. Publishing dissenting theories is important when they are backed by plausible evidence, but this does not mean giving critics 'equal time' to dissent from every finding by a mainstream scientist.

— Goertzel, 2010[56]

The HIV/AIDS denialist community[edit]

Denialists often use their critique of the link between HIV and AIDS to promote underline alternative medicine as a cure, and attempt to convince HIV-infected individuals to avoid ARV therapy in favour of vitamins, massage, yoga and other unproven treatments.[57] Despite this promotion, denialists will often downplay any association with alternative therapies, and attempt to portray themselves as "dissidents". An article in the *Skeptical Inquirer* stated:

AIDS denialists [prefer] to characterize themselves as brave "dissidents" attempting to engage a hostile medical/industrial establishment in genuine scientific "debate." They complain that their attempts to raise questions and pose alternative hypotheses have been unjustly rejected or ignored at the cost of scientific progress itself...Given their resistance to all evidence to the contrary, today's AIDS dissidents are more aptly referred to as AIDS denialists.[57]

Several scientists have been associated with HIV/AIDS denialism, although they have not themselves studied AIDS or HIV.[9] One of the most famous and influential is Peter Duesberg, professor of molecular and cell biology at the University of California, Berkeley, who since 1987 has disputed that the scientific evidence shows that HIV causes AIDS.[21] Other scientists associated with HIV/AIDS denialism include biochemists David Rasnick and Harvey Bialy. Kary Mullis, who was awarded a Nobel Prize for his role in the development of PCR, has expressed sympathy for denialist theories.[58] Biologist Lynn Margulis argued that "there's no evidence that HIV is an infectious virus" and that AIDS symptoms "overlap...completely" with those of syphilis.[59] Pathologist Etienne de Harven also expressed sympathy for HIV/AIDS denial.[60][61]

Additional notable HIV/AIDS denialists include Australian

academic ethicist <u>Hiram Caton</u>, the late mathematician <u>Serge Lang</u>,[62] former college administrator <u>Henry Bauer</u>, journalist <u>Celia Farber</u>, American talk radio host and author on alternative and complementary medicine and nutrition <u>Gary Null</u>, and the late activist <u>Christine Maggiore</u>, who encouraged HIV-positive mothers to forgo anti-HIV treatment and whose 3-year-old daughter died of complications of untreated AIDS.[63] <u>Nate Mendel</u>, bassist with the rock band <u>Foo Fighters</u>, expressed support for HIV/AIDS denialist ideas and organized a benefit concert in January 2000 for Maggiore's organization <u>Alive & Well AIDS Alternatives</u>.[64] Organizations of HIV/AIDS denialists include the <u>Perth Group</u>, composed of several Australian hospital workers, and the Immunity Resource Foundation.[65]

HIV/AIDS denialism has received some support from <u>political conservatives</u> in the United States. Duesberg's work has been published in *Policy Review*, a journal once published by the <u>Heritage Foundation</u> but now owned by the <u>Hoover Institution</u>,[66][67][68] and by <u>Regnery Press</u>,[69] as has journalist <u>Tom Bethell</u>'s book *The Politically Incorrect Guide to Science*, which endorses HIV/AIDS denialism.[70] Law professor <u>Phillip E. Johnson</u> has accused the <u>Centers for Disease Control</u> of "fraud" in relation to HIV/AIDS.[71] Describing the political aspects of the HIV/AIDS denialism movement, <u>Sociology</u> professor <u>Steven Epstein</u> wrote in *Impure Science* that "... the appeal of Duesberg's views to conservatives—certainly including those with little sympathy for the gay movement—cannot be denied."[66] The blog LewRockwell.com has also published articles supportive of HIV/AIDS denialism.[72]

In a follow-up article in *Skeptical Inquirer*,[73] Nattrass overviewed the prominent members of the HIV/AIDS denialist community and discussed the reasons of the intractable staying power of HIV/AIDS denialism in spite of scientific and medical consensus supported by over two decades of evidence. She observed that despite being a disparate group of people with very different background and professions, the HIV/AIDS denialists self-organize to fill four important roles:[73]

- Hero scientists to provide scientific legitimacy: Most notably is Peter Duesberg who plays the central role of HIV/AIDS denialism from the beginning. Others include David Rasnick, Etienne de Harven, and Kary Mullis whose Nobel Prize makes him symbolically important.
- "Cultropreneurs" to offer fake cures in place of antiretroviral therapy: Matthias Rath, Gary Null, Michael Ellner, and Roberto Giraldo all promote alternative medicine and remedies with a dose of conspiracy theories in the form of books, healing products, radio shows and counseling services.
- HIV positive living icons to provide proof of concept by appearing to live healthily without antiretroviral therapy: Christine Maggiore was and still is the most important icon in the HIV/AIDS denialist movement despite the fact that she died of AIDS related complications in 2008.
- Praise singers: sympathetic journalists and filmmakers who publicize the movement with uncritical and favorable opinion. They include journalists Celia Farber, Liam Scheff and Neville Hodgkinson; filmmakers Brent Leung and Robert Leppo.

Some of them had overlapping roles as board members of Rethinking AIDS and Alive and Well AIDS Alternatives, were involved in the film *House of Numbers*, *The Other Side of AIDS* or on Thabo Mbeki's AIDS Advisory Panel. Nattrass argued that HIV/AIDS denialism gains social traction through powerful community-building effects where these four organized characters from "a symbiotic connection between AIDS denialism and alternative healing modalities" and they are "facilitated by a shared conspiratorial stance toward HIV science".[73]

Former denialists [edit]

Several of the few prominent scientists who once voiced doubts about HIV/AIDS have since changed their views and accepted the fact that HIV plays a role in causing AIDS, in response to an accumulation of newer studies and data.[74] Robert Root-Bernstein, author of *Rethinking AIDS: The Tragic Cost of Premature Consensus* and formerly a critic of the causative role of HIV in AIDS, has since distanced himself from the HIV/AIDS denialist movement, saying, "Both the camp that says HIV is a pussycat and the people who claim AIDS is all HIV are wrong...The denialists make claims that are clearly inconsistent with existing studies."[75]

Joseph Sonnabend, who until the late 1990s regarded the issue of AIDS causation as unresolved, has reconsidered in light of the success of newer antiretroviral drugs, stating, "The evidence now strongly supports a role for HIV... Drugs that can save your life can also under different circumstances kill you. This is a distinction that denialists do not seem to understand."[75] Sonnabend has also criticized HIV/AIDS denialists for falsely implying that he supports their position, saying:

Some individuals who believe that HIV plays no role at all in AIDS have implied that I support their misguided views on AIDS causation by including inappropriate references to me in their literature and on their web sites. Before HIV was discovered and its association with AIDS established, I held the entirely appropriate view that the cause of AIDS was then unknown. I have successfully treated hundreds of AIDS patients with antiretroviral medications, and have no doubt that HIV plays a necessary role in this disease.[76]

Both Sonnabend and Root-Bernstein now favor a less controversial hypothesis, suggesting that while HIV is necessary for AIDS, cofactors may also contribute.

A former denialist wrote in the *Journal of Medical Ethics* in 2004:

The group [of denialists] regularly points to a substantial number of scientists supportive of its agenda to re-evaluate the HIV/AIDS hypothesis. Some of those members still listed are people who have been dead for a number of years. While it is correct that these people supported the objective of a scientific re-evaluation of the HIV/AIDS link when they were alive, it is clearly difficult to ascertain what these people would have made of the scientific developments and the accumulation of evidence for HIV as the crucial causative agent in AIDS, which has occurred in the years after their deaths.[55]

Death of HIV-positive denialists[edit]

In 2007, aidstruth.org, a website run by HIV researchers to counter denialist claims,[77] published a partial list of HIV/AIDS denialists who had died of AIDS-related causes. For example, the editors of the magazine _Continuum_ consistently denied the existence of HIV/AIDS. The magazine shut down when its editors all died of AIDS-related causes.[78] In each case, the HIV/AIDS denialist community attributed the deaths to unknown causes, secret drug use, or stress rather than HIV/AIDS.[19][55] Similarly, several HIV-positive former dissidents have reported being ostracized by the AIDS-denialist community after they developed AIDS and decided to pursue effective antiretroviral treatment.[79]

In 2008, activist Christine Maggiore died at the age of 52 while under a doctor's care for pneumonia. Maggiore, mother of two children, had founded an organisation to help other HIV-positive mothers avoid taking antiretroviral drugs that reduce the risk of HIV transmission from mother to child.[80] After her three-year-old daughter died of AIDS-related pneumonia in 2005, Maggiore continued to believe that HIV is not the cause of AIDS, and she and her husband Robin Scovill sued Los Angeles County and others on behalf of their daughter's estate, for allegedly violating Eliza Scovill's civil rights by releasing an autopsy report that listed her cause of death as AIDS-related pneumonia.[63] The litigants settled out of court, with the county paying Scovill $15,000 in March 2009, with no admission of wrongdoing. The L.A. coroner's ruling that Eliza Jane Scovill died of AIDS remains standing as the official verdict.[81]

Impact beyond the scientific community[edit]

AIDS-denialist claims have failed to attract support in the scientific community, where the evidence for the causative role of HIV in AIDS is considered conclusive. However, the movement has had a significant impact in the political sphere, culminating with former South African President Thabo Mbeki's embrace of AIDS-denialist claims.[82] The resulting governmental refusal to provide effective anti-HIV treatment in South Africa has been blamed for hundreds of thousands of premature AIDS-related deaths in South Africa.[44]

Impact in North America and Europe[edit]

Skepticism about HIV being the cause of AIDS began almost immediately after the discovery of HIV was announced. One of the earliest prominent skeptics was the journalist John Lauritsen, who argued in his writings for the *New York Native* that AIDS was in fact caused by amyl nitrite poppers, and that the government had conspired to hide the truth.[83]

In the scientific literature[edit]

The publication of Peter Duesberg's first AIDS paper in 1987 provided visibility for denialist claims. Shortly afterwards, the journal *Science* reported that Duesberg's remarks had won him "a large amount of media attention, particularly in the gay press where he is something of a hero."[84] However, Duesberg's support in the gay community dried up as he made a series of statements perceived as homophobic; in an interview with the *Village Voice* in 1988, Duesberg stated his belief that the AIDS epidemic was "caused by a lifestyle that was criminal twenty years ago."[85]

In the following few years, others became skeptical of the HIV theory as researchers initially failed to produce an effective treatment or vaccine for AIDS.[86] Journalists such as Neville Hodgkinson and Celia Farber regularly promoted denialist ideas in the American and British media; several television documentaries were also produced to increase awareness of the alternative viewpoint.[87] In 1992–1993, *The Sunday Times*, where

Hodgkinson served as scientific editor, ran a series of articles arguing that the AIDS epidemic in Africa was a myth. These articles stressed Duesberg's claims and argued that antiviral therapy was ineffective, HIV testing unreliable, and that AIDS was not a threat to heterosexuals. The *Sunday Times* coverage was heavily criticized as slanted, misleading, and potentially dangerous; the scientific journal *Nature* took the unusual step of printing a 1993 editorial calling the paper's coverage of HIV/AIDS "seriously mistaken, and probably disastrous."[88]

Finding difficulty in publishing his arguments in the scientific literature, Duesberg exercised his right as a member of the National Academy of Sciences to publish in *Proceedings of the National Academy of Sciences of the United States of America* (*PNAS*) without going through the peer review process. However, Duesberg's paper raised a "red flag" at the journal and was submitted by the editor for non-binding review. All of the reviewers found major flaws in Duesberg's paper; the reviewer specifically chosen by Duesberg noted the presence of "misleading arguments", "nonlogical statements", "misrepresentations", and political overtones.[25] Ultimately, the editor of *PNAS* acquiesced to publication,[89] writing to Duesberg: "If you wish to make these unsupported, vague, and prejudicial statements in print, so be it. But I cannot see how this would be convincing to any scientifically trained reader."[25]

HIV/AIDS denialists often resort to special pleading to support their assertion, arguing for different causes of AIDS in different locations and subpopulations. In North America, AIDS is blamed on the health effects of unprotected anal sex and poppers on homosexual men, an argument which does not account for AIDS in drug-free heterosexual women who deny participating in anal sex. In this case, HIV/AIDS denialists claim the women are having anal sex but refuse to disclose it. In haemophiliac North American children who contracted AIDS from blood transfusions, the haemophilia itself or its treatment is claimed to cause AIDS. In Africa, AIDS is blamed on poor nutrition and sanitation due to poverty. For wealthy populations in South Africa with adequate nutrition and sanitation, it is claimed that the antiretroviral drugs used to treat AIDS cause the condition. In each case, the <u>most parsimonious explanation</u> and uniting factor – HIV positive status – is ignored, as are the thousands of studies that converge on the common conclusion that AIDS is caused by HIV infection.[5]

Haemophilia is considered the best test of the HIV-AIDS hypothesis by both denialists and scientists. While Duesberg claims AIDS in haemophiliacs is caused by contaminated clotting factors and HIV is a harmless <u>passenger virus</u>, this result is contradicted by large studies on haemophiliac patients who received contaminated blood. A comparison of groups receiving high, medium and low levels of contaminated clotting factors found the death rates differed significantly depending on HIV status. Of 396 HIV positive haemophiliacs followed between 1985 and 1993, 153 died. The comparative figure for the HIV negative group was one out of 66, despite comparable doses of contaminated clotting factors. A comparison of individuals receiving blood donations also supports the results; in 1994 there were 6888 individuals with AIDS who had their HIV infection traced to blood transfusions. Since the introduction of HIV testing, the number of individuals whose AIDS status can be traced to blood transfusions was only 29 (as of 1994).[4]

In lay press and on the Internet[edit]

With the introduction of <u>highly active antiretroviral therapy</u> (HAART) in 1996–1997, the survival and general health of people with HIV improved significantly.[54][90] The positive response to treatment with anti-HIV medication cemented the scientific acceptance of the HIV/AIDS paradigm, and led several prominent HIV/AIDS denialists to accept the causative role of HIV.[55][75] Finding their arguments increasingly discredited by the scientific community, denialists took their message to the popular press. A former denialist wrote:

Scientists among the HIV dissidents used their academic credentials and academic affiliations to generate interest, sympathy, and allegiances in lay audiences. They were not professionally troubled about recruiting lay people—who were clearly unable to evaluate the scientific validity or otherwise of their views—to their cause.[55]

In addition to elements of the popular and alternative press, AIDS denialist ideas are propagated largely via the Internet.[91]

A 2007 article in *PLoS Medicine* noted:

Because these denialist assertions are made in books and on the Internet rather than in the scientific literature, many scientists are either unaware of the existence of organized denial groups, or believe they can safely ignore them as the discredited fringe. And indeed, most of the HIV deniers' arguments were answered long ago by scientists. However, many members of the general public do not have the scientific background to critique the assertions put forth by these groups, and not only accept them but continue to propagate them.[8]

AIDS activists have expressed concern that denialist arguments about HIV's harmlessness may be responsible for an upsurge in HIV infections. Denialist claims continue to exert a significant influence in some communities; a survey conducted at minority gay pride events in four American cities in 2005 found that 33% of attendees doubted that HIV caused AIDS.[92] According to Stephen Thomas, director of the University of Pittsburgh Center for Minority Health, "people are focusing on the wrong thing. They're focusing on conspiracies rather than protecting themselves, rather than getting tested and seeking out appropriate care and treatment."[93]

Impact in South Africa[edit]

Main article: HIV/AIDS denialism in South Africa

HIV/AIDS denialist claims have had a major political, social, and public health impact in South Africa. The government of then President Thabo Mbeki was sympathetic to the views of

HIV/AIDS denialists, with critics charging that denialist influence was responsible for the slow and ineffective governmental response to the country's massive AIDS epidemic.

Independent studies have arrived at almost identical estimates of the human costs of HIV/AIDS denialism in South Africa. According to a paper written by researchers from the Harvard School of Public Health, between 2000 and 2005, more than 330,000 deaths and an estimated 35,000 infant HIV infections occurred "because of a failure to accept the use of available [antiretroviral drugs] to prevent and treat HIV/AIDS in a timely manner."[13] Nicoli Nattrass of the University of Cape Town estimates that 343,000 excess AIDS deaths and 171,000 infections resulted from the Mbeki administration's policies, an outcome she refers to in the words of Peter Mandelson as "genocide by sloth".[14]

Durban Declaration[edit]

In 2000, when the International AIDS Conference was held in Durban, Mbeki convened a Presidential Advisory Panel containing a number of HIV/AIDS denialists, including Peter Duesberg and David Rasnick.[94] The Advisory Panel meetings were closed to the general press; an invited reporter from the *Village Voice* wrote that Rasnick advocated that HIV testing be legally banned and denied that he had seen "any evidence" of an AIDS catastrophe in South Africa, while Duesberg "gave a presentation so removed from African medical reality that it left several local doctors shaking their heads."[43]

In his address to the International AIDS Conference, Mbeki reiterated his view that HIV was not wholly responsible for AIDS, leading hundreds of delegates to walk out on his speech.[95] Mbeki also sent a letter to a number of world leaders likening the mainstream AIDS research community to supporters of the apartheid regime.[94] The tone and content of Mbeki's letter led diplomats in the U.S. to initially question whether it was a hoax.[96][97]

AIDS scientists and activists were dismayed at the president's behavior and responded with the Durban Declaration, a document affirming that HIV causes AIDS, signed by over 5,000 scientists and physicians.[112][95]

Criticism of governmental response[edit]

The former South African health minister Manto Tshabalala-Msimang also attracted heavy criticism, as she often promoted nutritional remedies such as garlic, lemons, beetroot and olive oil, to people suffering from AIDS,[98][99][100] while emphasizing possible toxicities of antiretroviral drugs, which she has referred to as "poison".[101] The South African Medical Association has accused Tshabalala-Msimang of "confusing a vulnerable public".[102] In September 2006, a group of over 80 scientists and academics called for "the immediate removal of Dr. Tshabalala-Msimang as minister of health and for an end to the disastrous, pseudoscientific policies that have characterized the South African government's response to HIV/AIDS."[103] In December 2006, deputy health minister Nozizwe Madlala-Routledge described "denial at the very highest levels" over AIDS.[104] She was subsequently fired by Mbeki.[105]

Former South African president Thabo Mbeki's government was widely criticized for delaying the rollout of programs to provide antiretroviral drugs to people with advanced HIV disease and to HIV-positive pregnant women. The national treatment program began only after the Treatment Action Campaign (TAC) brought a legal case against Government ministers, claiming they were responsible for the deaths of 600 HIV-positive people a day who could not access medication.[94][106] South Africa was one of the last countries in the region to begin such a treatment program, and roll-out has been much slower than planned.[101]

At the XVI International AIDS Conference, Stephen Lewis, UN special envoy for AIDS in Africa, attacked Mbeki's government for its slow response to the AIDS epidemic and reliance on denialist claims:

It [South Africa] is the only country in Africa … whose government is still obtuse, dilatory and negligent about rolling out treatment… It is the only country in Africa whose government continues to promote theories more worthy of a lunatic fringe than of a concerned and compassionate state.[103]

In 2002, Mbeki requested that HIV/AIDS denialists no longer use his name in denialist literature, and requested that denialists stop signing documents with "Member of President Mbeki's AIDS Advisory Panel".[94] This coincided with the South African government's statement accompanying its 2002 AIDS campaign, that "...in conducting this campaign, government's starting point is based on the premise that HIV causes AIDS".[107] Nonetheless, Mbeki himself continued to promote and defend AIDS-denialist claims. His loyalists attacked former President Nelson Mandela in 2002 when Mandela questioned the government's AIDS policy, and Mbeki attacked Malegapuru Makgoba, one of South Africa's leading scientists, as a racist defender of "Western science" for opposing HIV/AIDS denialism.[44]

In early 2005, former South African president Nelson Mandela announced that his son had died of complications of AIDS. Mandela's public announcement was seen as both an effort to combat the stigma associated with AIDS, and as a "political statement designed to… force the President [Mbeki] out of his denial."[108][109]

Post Mbeki government in South Africa[edit]

In 2008, Mbeki was ousted from power and replaced as President of South Africa by Kgalema Motlanthe. On Motlanthe's first day in office, he removed Manto Tshabalala-Msimang, the controversial health minister who had promoted AIDS-denialist claims and recommended garlic, beetroot, and lemon juice as treatments for AIDS. Barbara Hogan, newly appointed as health minister, voiced shame at the Mbeki government's embrace of HIV/AIDS denialism and vowed a new course, stating: "The era of denialism is over completely in South Africa."[44]

See also[edit]

- Misconceptions about HIV and AIDS
- Discredited HIV/AIDS origins theories
- *The Other Side of AIDS* (documentary film)
- "Retro" - the October 28, 2008 episode of the TV series *Law & Order: Special Victims Unit*, which focuses on an AIDS denialist doctor and the HIV-positive patients he has influenced.
- Denial (Psychology)

Footnotes[edit]

1.   ^ Jump up to: *a b c d* "Confronting AIDS: Update 1988". Institute of Medicine of the U.S. National Academy of Sciences. 1988. "...the evidence that HIV causes AIDS is scientifically conclusive."

2.   ^ Jump up to: *a b c d e f g* "The Evidence that HIV Causes AIDS". National Institute of Allergy and Infectious Disease. 4 September 2009. Retrieved 14 October 2009.

3.   **Jump up** ^ Kalichman 2009, p. 205.

4.   ^ Jump up to: *a b* Cohen, J. (1994). "Duesberg and critics agree: hemophilia is the best test". *Science* **266** (5191): 1645–1646. Bibcode:1994Sci...266.1645C. doi:10.1126/science.7992044. PMID 7992044. edit

5.   ^ Jump up to: *a b* Kalichman 2009.

6.   ^ Jump up to: *a b c* Cohen, J. (1994). "The Duesberg phenomenon". *Science* **266** (5191): 1642–1644. Bibcode:1994Sci...266.1642C. doi:10.1126/science.7992043. PMID 7992043. edit

7.   **Jump up** ^ "Denying science". *Nat. Med.* **12** (4): 369. 2006. doi:10.1038/nm0406-369. PMID 16598265. "To support their ideas, some AIDS denialists have also misappropriated a scientific review in *Nature Medicine* which opens with this reasonable statement: "Despite considerable advances in HIV science in the past 20 years, the reason why HIV-1 infection is pathogenic is still debated.""

8.   ^ Jump up to: *a b c* Smith, TC; Novella, SP (August 2007). "HIV denial in the internet era". *PLOS Medicine* **4** (8): e256. doi:10.1371/journal.pmed.0040256. PMC 1949841. PMID 17713982. Archived from the original on 6 May 2008.

9.   ^ Jump up to: *a b* Steinberg, J (17 June 2009). "AIDS denial: A lethal delusion". *New Scientist* **2713**. Retrieved 14 October 2009.

10. **Jump up** ^ Watson J. (2006). "Scientists, activists sue South Africa's AIDS 'denialists'". *Nat Med.* **12** (1): 6. doi:10.1038/nm0106-6a. PMID 16397537.

11. **Jump up** ^ Boseley, S (14 May 2005). "Discredited doctor's 'cure' for Aids ignites life-and-death struggle in South Africa". *The Guardian* (London). Retrieved 14 October 2009.

12. ^ Jump up to: *a b c* , (2000). "The Durban Declaration". *Nature* **406** (6791): 15–6. doi:10.1038/35017662. PMID 10894520.

13. ^ Jump up to: *a b c* Chigwedere P, Seage GR, Gruskin S, Lee TH, Essex M (October 2008). "Estimating the Lost Benefits of Antiretroviral Drug Use in South Africa". *Journal of acquired immune deficiency syndromes (1999)* **49** (4): 410–415. doi:10.1097/QAI.0b013e31818a6cd5. PMID 19186354. Lay summary.

14. ^ Jump up to: *a b c* Nattrass N (February 2008). "Estimating the Lost Benefits of Antiretroviral Drug Use in South Africa". *African Affairs* **107** (427): 157–76. doi:10.1093/afraf/adm087.

15. **Jump up** ^ Barré-Sinoussi, F; Chermann, J; Rey, F; Nugeyre, M; Chamaret, S; Gruest, J; Dauguet, C; Axler-Blin, C; Vézinet-Brun, F; Rouzioux, C; Rozenbaum, W; Montagnier, L (1983). "Isolation of a T-lymphotropic retrovirus from a patient at risk for acquired immune deficiency syndrome (AIDS)". *Science* **220** (4599): 868–71. Bibcode:1983Sci...220..868B. doi:10.1126/science.6189183. PMID 6189183.

16. **Jump up** ^ Sarngadharan, MG; DeVico, AL; Bruch, L; Schüpbach, J; Gallo, RC (1984). "HTLV-III: The etiologic agent of AIDS". *Int. Symp. Princess Takamatsu Cancer Res. Fund* **15**: 301–8. PMID 6100648.

17. **Jump up** ^ Schmidt, C (1984). "The group-fantasy origins of AIDS". *Journal of Psychohistory* **12** (1): 37–78. PMID 11611586.

18. **Jump up** ^ Kalichman 2009, p. 26.

19. ^ Jump up to: *a b* "AIDS Denialists Who Have Died". *aidstruth.org*. Retrieved 15 June 2009.

20. **Jump up** ^ Coffin, J; Haase, A; Levy, J; Montagnier, L; Oroszlan, S; Teich, N; Temin, H; Toyoshima, K; Varmus, H; Vogt, P (1986). "What to call the AIDS virus?". *Nature* **321** (6065): 10. Bibcode:1986Natur.321...10.. doi:10.1038/321010a0. PMID 3010128.

21. ^ Jump up to: *a b* Duesberg, P (1987). "Retroviruses as carcinogens and pathogens: Expectations and reality". *Cancer Research* **47** (5): 1199–220. PMID 3028606.

22. **Jump up** ^ Blattner, W; Gallo, RC; Temin, HM (1988). "HIV causes AIDS". *Science* **241** (4865): 515–6. Bibcode:1988Sci...241..515B. doi:10.1126/science.3399881. PMID 3399881.

23. **Jump up** ^ Duesberg, P (1988). "HIV is not the cause of AIDS". *Science* **241** (4865): 514. Bibcode:1988Sci...241..514D. doi:10.1126/science.3399880. PMID 3399880.

24.   **Jump up** ^ Papadopulos-Eleopulos, E (1988). "Reappraisal of AIDS – Is the oxidation induced by the risk factors the primary cause?". *Medical Hypotheses* **25** (3): 151–62. doi:10.1016/0306-9877(88)90053-9. PMID 3285143.

25.   ^ Jump up to: *a* *b* *c* Booth, W (1989). "AIDS paper raises red flag at PNAS". *Science* **243** (4892): 733. Bibcode:1989Sci...243..733B. doi:10.1126/science.2916121. PMID 2916121.

26.   **Jump up** ^ Root-Bernstein, R (1990). "Do we know the cause(s) of AIDS?". *Perspectives in Biology and Medicine* **33** (4): 480–500. PMID 2216658.

27.   **Jump up** ^ Maddox, J (1993). "Has Duesberg a right of reply?". *Nature* **363** (6425): 109. Bibcode:1993Natur.363..109M. doi:10.1038/363109a0. PMID 8483492.

28.   ^ Jump up to: *a* *b* Papadopulos-Eleopulos, E; Turner, VF; Papadimitriou, JM (1993). "Is a positive western blot proof of HIV infection?". *Nature Biotechnology* **11** (6): 696–707. doi:10.1038/nbt0693-696. PMID 7763673.

29.   **Jump up** ^ Kalichman 2009, p. 170.

30.   **Jump up** ^ Bugl, P. "The Rise of HIV/AIDS". Department of Mathematics, University of Hartford. Archived from the original on 4 February 2007. Retrieved 22 January 2007.

31.   **Jump up** ^ Baumann, E; Bethell, T; Bialy, H; Duesberg, P; Farber, C; Geshekter, C; Johnson, P; Maver, R; Schoch, R; Stewart, G (1995). "AIDS proposal. Group for the Scientific Reappraisal of the HIV/AIDS Hypothesis". *Science* **267** (5200): 945–6. Bibcode:1995Sci...267..945B. doi:10.1126/science.267.5200.945. PMID 7863335.

32.   ^ Jump up to: *a* *b* King, E (1996). "Isolated facts about HIV: A response to claims by AIDS dissidents that HIV doesn't exist". *AIDS Treatment Update* **40**.

33.   **Jump up** ^ Sabin, CA; Phillips, AN; Lee, CA (1996). "Response: Arguments contradict the "foreign protein-zidovudine" hypothesis". *BMJ* **312** (7025): 211–2. doi:10.1136/bmj.312.7025.211. PMC 2350000. PMID 8563584.

34.   **Jump up** ^ Papadopulos-Eleopulos, E; Turner, VF; Papadimitriou, JM; Stewart, G; Causer, D (1997). "HIV antibodies: Further questions and a plea for clarification". *Current Medical Research and Opinion* **13** (10): 627–34. doi:10.1185/03007999709113336. PMID 9327197.

35.   **Jump up** ^ Papadopulos-Eleopulos, E; Turner, VF; Papadimitriou, JM; Causer, D; Page, BA (1998). "HIV antibody tests and viral load — More unanswered questions and a further plea for clarification". *Current Medical Research and Opinion* **14** (3): 185–6. doi:10.1185/03007999809113358. PMID 9787984.

36.   **Jump up** ^ Papadopulos-Eleopulos, E; Turner, VF; Page, BA; Papadimitriou, J; Causer, D (2006). "No proof HIV antibodies are

caused by a retroviral infection". Letters to the Editor. *Emergency Medicine Australasia* **18** (3): 308–10. doi:10.1111/j.1742-6723.2006.00859.x. PMID 16712545.

37.   **Jump up** ^ Farber, C (March 2006). "Out of control: AIDS and the corruption of medical science". *Harper's Magazine*. Archived from the original on 4 May 2009. Retrieved 11 June 2009.

38.   **Jump up** ^ Miller, L (13 March 2006). "An article in Harper's ignites a controversy over HIV". *The New York Times*. Retrieved 25 May 2008.

39.   **Jump up** ^ Gallo, R; Geffen, N; Gonsalves, G; Jefferys, R; Kuritzkes, DR; Mirken, B; Moore, JP; Safrit, JT (25 March 2006). "Errors in Celia Farber's March 2006 article in Harper's Magazine". Treatment Action Campaign. Archived from the original on 16 June 2009. Retrieved 11 June 2009.

40.   **Jump up** ^ "Shadow of doubters". *Brisbane Times*. 5 May 2007. Archived from the original on 27 April 2009. Retrieved 11 June 2009.

41.   **Jump up** ^ "Boy is healthy without drug for HIV, mother says". *The New York Times*. 20 September 1998. Retrieved 11 June 2009.

42.   **Jump up** ^ Harkavy, J (10 March 2006). "Nikolas Emerson, 11; Case led to legal fight over HIV". *Boston Globe*. Retrieved 11 June 2009.

43.   ^ Jump up to: *a b* Schoofs, M (5 July 2000). "Debating the obvious: Inside the South African government's controversial AIDS panel". *Village Voice*. Retrieved 11 June 2009.

44.   ^ Jump up to: *a b c d* Dugger, C (25 November 2008). "Study cites toll of AIDS policy in South Africa". *The New York Times*. Retrieved 17 December 2008.

45.   **Jump up** ^ Turner, V (1999). "E-Mail Correspondence Between Val Turner and Robin Weiss". *virusmyth.com*.

46.   **Jump up** ^ Duesberg, P (1989). "Human immunodeficiency virus and acquired immunodeficiency syndrome: Correlation but not causation". *Proceedings of the National Academy of Sciences of the United States of America* **86** (3): 755–64. Bibcode:1989PNAS...86..755D. doi:10.1073/pnas.86.3.755. PMC 286556. PMID 2644642.

47.   **Jump up** ^ "10 Scientific Reasons Why HIV Cannot Cause AIDS". *HealToronto.com*. Retrieved 28 September 2006.

48.   **Jump up** ^ Duesberg, P; Koehnlein, C; Rasnick, D (2003). "The chemical bases of the various AIDS epidemics: Recreational drugs, anti-viral chemotherapy and malnutrition". *Journal of Biosciences* **28** (4): 383–412. doi:10.1007/BF02705115. PMID 12799487.

49.   **Jump up** ^ "Basic Information about HIV and AIDS". Centers for Disease Control. 11 August 2010. Retrieved 4 February 2011.

50.   **Jump up** ^ O'Brien, SJ; Goedert, JJ (1996). "HIV causes AIDS: Koch's postulates fulfilled". *Current Opinion in Immunology* **8** (5): 613–8. doi:10.1016/S0952-7915(96)80075-6. PMID 8902385.

51.   **Jump up** ^ "HIV Science and Responsible Journalism". XVI International AIDS Conference. 13 August 2006. Retrieved 17 December 2008.

52.   **Jump up** ^ Moore, John (16 May 2008). "How Immunoassays Work: The Curious Case of AIDS Denialist Roberto Giraldo and his Ignorance of the Basics". Aidstruth.org. Retrieved 17 December 2008.

53.   **Jump up** ^ Steinberg, J (23 June 2009). "Five myths about HIV and AIDS". *New Scientist*. Retrieved 4 February 2011.

54.   ^ Jump up to: *a b* Major studies confirming the benefits and effectiveness of modern anti-HIV therapy include, but are not limited to:

- Lima V, Hogg R, Harrigan P, Moore D, Yip B, Wood E, Montaner J (2007). "Continued improvement in survival among HIV-infected individuals with newer forms of highly active antiretroviral therapy". *AIDS* **21** (6): 685–92. doi:10.1097/QAD.0b013e32802ef30c. PMID 17413689.

- Jordan R, Gold L, Cummins C, Hyde C (2002). "Systematic review and meta-analysis of evidence for increasing numbers of drugs in antiretroviral combination therapy". *BMJ* **324** (7340): 757. doi:10.1136/bmj.324.7340.757. PMC 100314. PMID 11923157.

- Ivers L, Kendrick D, Doucette K (2005). "Efficacy of antiretroviral therapy programs in resource-poor settings: a meta-analysis of the published literature". *Clin Infect Dis* **41** (2): 217–24. doi:10.1086/431199. PMID 15983918.

- Mocroft A, Ledergerber B, Katlama C, Kirk O, Reiss P, d'Arminio Monforte A, Knysz B, Dietrich M, Phillips A, Lundgren J (2003). "Decline in the AIDS and death rates in the EuroSIDA study: an observational study". *Lancet* **362** (9377): 22–9. doi:10.1016/S0140-6736(03)13802-0. PMID 12853195.

- Sterne J, Hernán M, Ledergerber B, Tilling K, Weber R, Sendi P, Rickenbach M, Robins J, Egger M (2005). "Long-term effectiveness of potent antiretroviral therapy in preventing AIDS and death: a prospective cohort study". *Lancet* **366** (9483): 378–84. doi:10.1016/S0140-6736(05)67022-5. PMID 16054937.

55.   ^ Jump up to: *a b c d e* Schüklenk, U (2004). "Professional responsibilities of biomedical scientists in public discourse". *J Med Ethics* **30** (1): 53–60; discussion 61–2. doi:10.1136/jme.2003.002980. PMC 1757140. PMID 14872076.

56.   ^ Jump up to: *a b* Goertzel, T. (2010). "Conspiracy theories in science". *EMBO Reports* **11** (7): 493–499. doi:10.1038/embor.2010.84. PMC 2897118. PMID 20539311. edit

57.   ^ Jump up to: *a b* Nattrass, N (2007). "AIDS Denialism vs. Science". *Skeptical Inquirer* **31** (5).

58.   **Jump up** ^ Mullis, K (1998). *Dancing Naked in the Mind Field*. Vintage Books. pp. 171–182. ISBN 0679442553.

59.   **Jump up** ^ Teresi, D (April 2011). "Lynn Margulis: Q & A". *Discover Magazine*. pp. 66–70. Archived from the original on 21 April 2011. Retrieved 14 April 2011.

60.   **Jump up** ^ Rohleder, P; Swartz, L; Kalichman, SC (2009). *HIV/AIDS in South Africa 25 years On: Psychosocial Perspectives*. Springer. p. 125. ISBN 9781441903051..

61.   **Jump up** ^ Kalichman 2009, pp. 61, 128, 180.

62.   **Jump up** ^ Chang, K; Leary, W (25 September 2005). "Serge Lang, 78, a gadfly and mathematical theorist, dies". *The New York Times*. Retrieved 23 April 2010.

63.   ^ Jump up to: *a b* Gorman, A; Zavis, A (30 December 2008). "Christine Maggiore, vocal skeptic of AIDS research, dies at 52". *Los Angeles Times*. Archived from the original on 31 December 2008. Retrieved 30 December 2008.

64.   **Jump up** ^ "Foo Fighters, HIV Deniers". *Mother Jones*. 25 February 2000. Archived from the original on 27 November 2006. Retrieved 21 October 2006.

65.   **Jump up** ^ "Immunity Resource Foundation (IRF)". IRF.

66.   ^ Jump up to: *a b* Epstein 1996, pp. 131–158.

67.   **Jump up** ^ Duesberg, P; Ellison, BJ (Summer 1990). "Is the AIDS virus a science fiction". *Policy Review*. pp. 40–51.

68.   **Jump up** ^ Duesberg, P; Ellison, BJ (Fall 1990). "Is HIV the cause of AIDS?". *Policy Review*. pp. 70–83.

69.   **Jump up** ^ Horton, R (23 May 1996). "Truth and heresy about AIDS". *The New York Review of Books*.

70.   **Jump up** ^ Bethell, T (2005). *The Politically Incorrect Guide to Science*. Regnery Publishing. pp. 105–122. ISBN 089526031X.

71.   **Jump up** ^ "HIV & AIDS – Statement About CDC Fraud". *virusmyth.com*. Retrieved 18 March 2008.

72.   **Jump up** ^ Kalichman 2009, pp. 50–53.

73.   ^ Jump up to: *a b c* Nattrass, N (July–August 2012). "The social and symbolic power of AIDS denialism". *Skeptical Inquirer* (Committee for Skeptical Inquiry) **36**: 34–8.

74. **Jump up** ^ Delaney, M (2005). "HIV, AIDS, and the distortion of science". *Focus* **15** (6). pp. 1–6. Archived from the original on 4 June 2011. Retrieved 9 June 2011.

75. ^ Jump up to: *a b c* Lederer, B (1 April 2006). "Dead Certain?". *POZ*. Archived from the original on 13 November 2006. Retrieved 31 October 2006.

76. **Jump up** ^ "Statement by Joseph Sonnabend, M.D.". *aidstruth.org*. Retrieved 15 February 2011.

77. **Jump up** ^ Cohen, J (2007). "HIV/AIDS. AIDSTruth.org Web site takes aim at 'denialists'". *Science* **316** (5831): 1554. doi:10.1126/science.316.5831.1554. PMID 17569834.

78. **Jump up** ^ Kalichman, S (November 2009). "How to spot an AIDS denialist". *New Humanist*.

79. **Jump up** ^ Mirken, B (2 February 2000). "Bad science: They once thought HIV was harmless. Now, they say, AIDS has forced them to reconsider". *San Francisco Bay Guardian*. Archived from the original on 15 April 2008. Retrieved 9 May 2008.

80. **Jump up** ^ Ornstein, C; Costello, D (24 September 2005). "A mother's denial, a daughter's death". *Los Angeles Times*. Archived from the original on 22 December 2008. Retrieved 29 December 2008.

81. **Jump up** ^ Hennessy-Fiske, M (6 March 2009). "Suit settled on autopsy of HIV skeptics' child". *The Los Angeles Times*.

82. **Jump up** ^ Gray, Adrian. "The Politics of AIDS Denialism: South Africa's Failure to Respond - By Pieter Fourie and Melissa Meyer". *Political Studies Review* **10** (2): 309–309. doi:10.1111/j.1478-9302.2012.00269_2.x.

83. **Jump up** ^ "Biography of John Lauritsen". *virusmyth.com*. Retrieved 7 September 2006.

84. **Jump up** ^ Booth, W (1988). "A rebel without a cause of AIDS". *Science* **239** (4847): 1485–8. Bibcode:1988Sci...239.1485B. doi:10.1126/science.3281251. PMID 3281251.

85. **Jump up** ^ Epstein, S (1996). *Impure Science: AIDS, Activism, and the Politics of Knowledge*. Berkeley: University of California Press. p. 118. ISBN 0520202333.

86. **Jump up** ^ Burkett, E (1996) The Gravest Show on Earth (Chapter 2) ISBN 0-312-14607-8

87. **Jump up** ^ "Censorship". *virusmyth.com*. Retrieved 2 June 2006.

88. **Jump up** ^ Schmidt, WE (10 December 1993). "British paper and science journal clash on AIDS". *The New York Times*. Retrieved 25 April 2008.

89. **Jump up** ^ Duesberg, PH (1989). "Human immunodeficiency virus and acquired immunodeficiency syndrome: Correlation but not causation". *Proceedings of the National Academy of Sciences of the United States of America* **86** (3): 755–64.

Bibcode:1989PNAS...86..755D. doi:10.1073/pnas.86.3.755. PMC 286556. PMID 2644642.

90.   **Jump up ^** May, M. T.; Sterne, J. A.; Costagliola, D.; Sabin, C. A.; Phillips, A. N.; Justice, A. C.; Dabis, F.; Gill, J.; Lundgren, J.; Hogg, R. S.; De Wolf, F.; Fätkenheuer, G.; Staszewski, S.; d'Arminio Monforte, A.; Egger, M.; Antiretroviral Therapy (ART) Cohort Collaboration (2006). "HIV treatment response and prognosis in Europe and North America in the first decade of highly active antiretroviral therapy: A collaborative analysis". *The Lancet* **368** (9534): 451–458. doi:10.1016/S0140-6736(06)69152-6. PMID 16890831. edit

91.   **Jump up ^** Deer, B (21 February 2012). "Death by denial: The campaigners who continue to deny HIV causes Aids". *The Guardian*.

92.   **Jump up ^** Hutchinson, AB; Begley, EB; et al. (2005). "Mistrust and conspiracy beliefs about HIV/AIDS among participants in minority gay pride events". *2005 National HIV Prevention Conference*: Abstract TP-011.

93.   **Jump up ^** France, D (19 August 2000). "The HIV Disbelievers". *Newsweek*.

94.   ^ Jump up to: *a b c d* "The Politics of HIV/AIDS in South Africa". *JournAIDS*. HIV & AIDS Media Project. Archived from the original on 2 July 2007. Retrieved 26 February 2007.

95.   ^ Jump up to: *a b* "Controversy dogs AIDS forum". *BBC News*. 10 July 2000. Retrieved 26 February 2007.

96.   **Jump up ^** Schoof, M (5–11 July 2000). "Proof positive: How African science has demonstrated that HIV causes AIDS". *Village Voice*. Retrieved 20 April 2007.

97.   **Jump up ^** Gellman, B (19 April 2000). "South African president escalates AIDS feud". *Washington Post*. Retrieved 26 February 2007. (subscription required (help)).

98.   **Jump up ^** Thom, A (21 August 2006). "Beetroot battle at world AIDS conference". *Health-e*. Retrieved 9 March 2007.

99.   **Jump up ^** "'Dr Beetroot' hits back at media over Aids exhibition". *Mail & Guardian*. Retrieved 20 September 2006.

100.   **Jump up ^** "Manto again angers AIDS activists". *AEGIS.com*. Retrieved 20 September 2006.

101.   ^ Jump up to: *a b* Nattrass, N. "AIDS, science and governance". *aidstruth.org*.[*dead link*]

102.   **Jump up ^** "SAMA calls for end to misrepresentation on treatment of AIDS" (Press release). South African Medical Association. 29 August 2006. Retrieved 12 March 2007.

103.   ^ Jump up to: *a b* Leonard, T (6 September 2006). "Scientists rip S. African AIDS policies". *Washington Post*. Retrieved 5 March 2007.

104.   **Jump up** ^ Bevan, S (12 November 2006). "African minister ends decade of denial over AIDS". *The Daily Telegraph* (London). Archived from the original on 25 February 2007. Retrieved 5 March 2007.

105.   **Jump up** ^ "Sacked S Africa minister hits out". *BBC News*. 10 August 2007. Retrieved 11 August 2007.

106.   **Jump up** ^ "Current Developments Preventing Mother-To-Child HIV Transmission In South Africa: Background, Strategies And Outcomes Of The Treatment Action Campaign Case Against The Minister Of Health".

107.   **Jump up** ^ "AIDS in South Africa: Treatment, transmission and the government". *avert.org*.

108.   **Jump up** ^ Robinson, S (9 January 2005). "No place for denial". *Time*. Retrieved 26 February 2007.

109.   **Jump up** ^ Happold, T (6 January 2005). "Mandela's eldest son dies of AIDS". *The Guardian*. Retrieved 9 March 2007.

References[edit]

- *Kalichman, Seth (2009). Denying AIDS: Conspiracy Theories, Pseudoscience, and Human Tragedy. New York: Copernicus Books (Springer Science+Business Media). ISBN 9780387794754.*

Further reading[edit]

- Fourie, P (2006). *The Political Management of HIV and AIDS in South Africa: One Burden Too Many?*. Palgrave Macmillan. ISBN 0230006671.
- Steinberg, J (23 June 2009). "Five myths about HIV and AIDS". *New Scientist*. Archived from the original on 2 January 2010. Retrieved 25 December 2009.
- Nicoli Nattrass: *The AIDS Conspiracy: Science Fights Back:* New York: Columbia University Press: 2012.

External links[edit]

- National Institute of Allergy and Infectious Diseases pages on the HIV-AIDS connection and evidence that HIV causes AIDS

- Series of articles in *Science* magazine examining denialist claims
- Avert.org: Evidence that HIV causes AIDS
- AidsTruth.org, an organization that advocates against AIDS denialism

An **HIV vaccine** is a vaccine which would either protect individuals who do not have HIV from contracting that virus, or otherwise may have a therapeutic effect for persons who have or later contract HIV/AIDS. Currently, there is no effective HIV vaccine but many research projects managing clinical trials seek to create one. There is evidence that a vaccine may be possible. Work with monoclonal antibodies (MAb) has shown or proven that the human body can defend itself against HIV, and certain individuals remain asymptomatic for decades after HIV infection. Potential candidates for antibodies and early stage results from clinical trials have been announced.

One HIV vaccine candidate which showed some efficacy was studied in RV 144, which was a trial in Thailand beginning in 2003 and first reporting a positive result in 2009. Many trials have shown no efficacy, including the STEP study and HVTN 505 trials.[1]

Contents

[hide]

Overview[edit]

The urgency of the search for a vaccine against HIV stems from the AIDS-related death toll of over 25 million people since 1981.[2] Indeed, in 2002, AIDS became the primary cause of mortality due to an infectious agent in Africa.[3]

Alternative medical treatments to a vaccine do exist. Highly active antiretroviral therapy (HAART) has been highly beneficial to many HIV-infected individuals since its introduction in 1996 when the protease inhibitor-based HAART initially became available. HAART allows the stabilization of the patient's symptoms and viremia, but they do not cure the patient of HIV, nor of the symptoms of AIDS. And, importantly, HAART does nothing to prevent the spread of HIV by people with undiagnosed infections. Introduction of safer sex measures to halt the spread of AIDS has proven difficult in the worst affected countries.

Therefore, an HIV vaccine is generally considered as the most likely, and perhaps the only way by which the AIDS pandemic can be halted. However, after over 20 years of research, HIV-1 remains a difficult target for a vaccine.

Difficulties in developing an HIV vaccine[edit]

In 1984, after the confirmation of the etiological agent of AIDS by scientists at the U.S. National Institutes of Health and the Pasteur Institute, the United States Health and Human Services Secretary Margaret Heckler declared that a vaccine would be available within two years.[4]

However, the classical vaccination approaches that have been successful in the control of various viral diseases by priming the adaptive immunity to recognize the viral envelope proteins have failed in the case of HIV-1. Some have stated that an HIV vaccine may not be possible without significant theoretical advances.[5]

There are a number of factors that cause development of an HIV vaccine to differ from the development of other classic vaccines:[6]

- Classic vaccines mimic natural immunity against reinfection generally seen in individuals recovered from infection; there are almost no recovered AIDS patients.
- Most vaccines protect against disease, not against infection; HIV infection may remain latent for long periods before causing AIDS.
- Most effective vaccines are whole-killed or live-attenuated organisms; killed HIV-1 does not retain antigenicity and the use of a live retrovirus vaccine raises safety issues.
- Most vaccines protect against infections that are infrequently encountered; HIV may be encountered daily by individuals at high risk.
- Most vaccines protect against infections through mucosal surfaces of the respiratory or gastrointestinal tract; the great majority of HIV infection is through the genital tract.

HIV structure[edit]

The epitopes of the viral envelope are more variable than those of many other viruses. Furthermore, the functionally important epitopes of the gp120 protein are masked by glycosylation, trimerisation and receptor-induced conformational changes making it difficult to block with neutralising antibodies.

The ineffectiveness of previously developed vaccines primarily stems from two related factors.

- First, HIV is highly mutable. Because of the virus' ability to rapidly respond to selective pressures imposed by the immune system, the population of virus in an infected individual typically evolves so that it can evade the two major arms of the adaptive immune system; humoral (antibody-mediated) and cellular (mediated by T cells) immunity.
- Second, HIV isolates are themselves highly variable. HIV can be categorized into multiple clades and subtypes with a high degree of genetic divergence. Therefore, the immune responses raised by any vaccine need to be broad enough to account for this variability. Any vaccine that lacks this breadth is unlikely to be effective.

The difficulties in stimulating a reliable antibody response has led to the attempts to develop a vaccine that stimulates a response by cytotoxic T-lymphocytes.[7][7][8][8]

Another response to the challenge has been to create a single peptide that contains the least variable components of all the known HIV strains.[9]

Animal model[edit]

The typical animal model for vaccine research is the monkey, often the macaque. Monkeys can be infected with SIV or the chimeric SHIV for research purposes. However, the well-proven route of trying to induce neutralizing antibodies by vaccination has stalled because of the great difficulty in stimulating antibodies that neutralise heterologous primary HIV isolates.[10] Some vaccines based on the virus envelope have protected chimpanzees or macaques from homologous virus challenge,[11] but in clinical trials, individuals who were immunised with similar constructs became infected after later exposure to HIV-1.[12]

There are some differences between SIV and HIV that may introduce challenges in the use of an animal model.[13]

As published on 27 November 2009 in Journal of Biology, there is a new animal model strongly resembling that of HIV in humans. Generalized immune activation as a direct result of activated CD4+ T cell killing - performed in mice allows new ways of testing HIV behaviour.[14][15]

NIAID-funded SIV research has shown that challenging monkeys with a cytomegalovirus (CMV)-based SIV vaccine results in containment of virus. Typically, virus replication and dissemination occurs within days after infection, whereas vaccine-induced T cell activation and recruitment to sites of viral replication takes weeks. Researchers hypothesized that vaccines designed to maintain activated effector memory T cells might impair viral replication at its earliest stage.[citation needed]

Clinical trials to date[edit]

Several vaccine candidates are in varying phases of clinical trials.

Phase I[edit]

Most initial approaches have focused on the HIV envelope protein. At least thirteen different gp120 and gp160 envelope candidates have been evaluated, in the US predominantly through the AIDS Vaccine Evaluation Group. Most research focused on gp120 rather than gp41/gp160, as the latter are generally more difficult to produce and did not initially offer any clear advantage over gp120 forms. Overall, they have been safe and immunogenic in diverse populations, have induced neutralizing antibody in nearly 100%

recipients, but rarely induced CD8+ cytotoxic T lymphocytes (CTL). Mammalian derived envelope preparations have been better inducers of neutralizing antibody than candidates produced in yeast and bacteria. Although the vaccination process involved many repeated "booster" injections, it was very difficult to induce and maintain the high anti-gp120 antibody titers necessary to have any hope of neutralizing an HIV exposure.

The availability of several recombinant canarypox vectors has provided interesting results that may prove to be generalizable to other viral vectors. Increasing the complexity of the canarypox vectors by inclusion of more genes/epitopes has increased the percent of volunteers that have detectable CTL to a greater extent than did increasing the dose of the viral vector. Importantly, CTLs from volunteers were able to kill peripheral blood mononuclear cells infected with primary isolates of HIV, suggesting that induced CTLs could have biological significance. In addition, cells from at least some volunteers were able to kill cells infected with HIV from other clades, though the pattern of recognition was not uniform among volunteers. Canarypox is the first candidate HIV vaccine that has induced cross-clade functional CTL responses. The first phase I trial of the candidate vaccine in Africa was launched early in 1999 with Ugandan volunteers. The study determined the extent to which Ugandan volunteers have CTL that are active against the subtypes of HIV prevalent in Uganda, A and D.

Other strategies that have progressed to phase I trials in uninfected persons include peptides, lipopeptides, DNA, an attenuated Salmonella vector, p24, etc. Specifically, candidate vaccines that induce one or more of the following are being sought:

- neutralizing antibodies active against a broad range of HIV primary isolates;
- cytotoxic T cell responses in a vast majority of recipients;
- strong mucosal immune responses.

In 2011, researchers in National Biotech Centre in Madrid unveiled data from the Phase I clinical trial of their new vaccine, MVA-B. The vaccine was effective in inducing an immunological response in 92% of the healthy subjects.[16]

Phase II[edit]

On December 13, 2004, the HIV Vaccine Trials Network (HVTN) began recruiting for the STEP study, a 3,000-participant phase II clinical trial of a novel HIV vaccine, at sites in North America, South America, the Caribbean and Australia.[17] The trial was co-funded by the National Institute of Allergy and Infectious Diseases (NIAID), which is a division of the National Institutes of Health (NIH), and the pharmaceutical company Merck & Co. Merck developed the experimental vaccine called V520 to stimulate HIV-specific cellular immunity, which prompts the body to produce T cells that kill HIV-infected cells. In previous smaller trials, this vaccine was found to be safe, because of the lack of adverse effects on the patients. The vaccine showed induced cellular immune responses against HIV in more than half of volunteers.[2]

V520 contains a weakened adenovirus that serves as a carrier for three subtype B HIV genes (*gag* / *pol* / *nef*). Subtype B is the most prevalent HIV subtype in the regions of the study sites. Adenoviruses are among the main causes of upper respiratory tract ailments such as the common cold. Because the vaccine contains only three HIV genes housed in a weakened adenovirus, study participants cannot become infected with HIV or get a respiratory infection from the vaccine. It was announced in September 2007 that the trial for V520 would be discontinued after it determined that the vaccination appeared associated with an increased risk of HIV infection in some recipients.[18] The foremost issue facing the rAd5 adenovirus that was used is the high prevalence of the adenovirus-specific antibodies as a result of prior exposure to the virus. Adenovirus vectors and many other viral vectors currently used in HIV vaccines, will induce a rapid memory immune response against the vector. This results in an impediment to the development of a T cell response against the inserted antigen (HIV antigens)[19] Additionally, it appears that V520 may have made some recipients more receptive to infection by HIV-1.[20][21]

The HVTN expected to finish the study in 2009, but ceased further treatment administration and declared the vaccine ineffective at preventing HIV-infection in September 2007.[22] The results of the trial have caused some to call for a reexamination of vaccine development strategies.[23]

Phase III[edit]

In February 2003, VaxGen announced that their AIDSVAX vaccine was a failure in North America as there was not a statistically significant reduction of HIV infection within the study population. This same vaccine was retested in Thailand within a vaccine regimen called RV 144 beginning in 2003, with positive results. In both cases the vaccines targeted gp120 and were specific for the geographical regions. The Thai trial was the largest AIDS vaccine trial to date when it started.[24]

In October 2009, the results of the RV 144 trial were published. Initial results, released in September 2009 prior to publication of complete results, were encouraging for scientists in search of a vaccine. The study involved 16,395 participants who did not have HIV infection, 8197 of whom were given treatment consisting of two experimental vaccines targeting HIV types B and E that are prevalent in Thailand, while 8198 were given a placebo. The participants were tested for HIV every six months for three years. After three years, the vaccine group saw HIV infection rates reduced by more than 30% compared with those in the placebo group. However, after taking into account the seven people who had HIV infections at the time of their vaccination (two in the placebo group, five in the vaccine group) the percentage dropped to 26%.[24][25]

Further analysis presented at a 2011 AIDS conference in Bangkok revealed that participants receiving vaccines in the RV 144 trial who produced IgG antibodies against the V2 loop of the HIV outer envelope were 43% less likely to become infected than those who did not, while IgA production was associated with a 54% greater risk of infection than those who did not produce the antibodies (but not worse than placebo). Viruses collected from vaccinated participants possessed mutations in the V2 region. Tests of a vaccine for SIV in monkeys found greater resistance to SIV in animals producing antibodies against this region. For these reasons further vaccine development was expected to focus heavily on vaccines designed to provoke an IgG reaction against the V2 loop.[26]

Planned clinical trials[edit]

Novel approaches, including modified vaccinia Ankara (MVA), adeno-associated virus, Venezuelan equine encephalitis (VEE) replicons, and codon-optimized DNA have proven to be strong inducers of CTL in macaque models, and have provided at least partial protection in some models. Most of these approaches are in, or will soon enter, clinical studies.

Economics of vaccine development[edit]

A July 2012 report of the HIV Vaccines & Microbicides Resource Tracking Working Group estimates that $845 million was spent on AIDS vaccine research in 2011.[27]

Economic issues with developing an AIDS vaccine include the need for advance purchase commitment (or advance market commitments) because after an AIDS vaccine has been developed, governments and NGOs may be able to bid the price down to marginal cost.[28]

Classification of all theoretically possible HIV vaccines[edit]

Any theoretically possible HIV vaccines must inhibit or stop the HIV virion replication cycle.[29] So, the targets of the vaccine are the following phases of the HIV virion cycle:

- Phase I. Free state
- Phase II. Attachment
- Phase III. Penetration
- Phase IV. Uncoating
- Phase V. Replication
- Phase VI. Assembling
- Phase VII. Releasing

So, the possible approaches for the HIV vaccine are the following (in the bracket specified the *Phases* were it is possible to do).

Filtering virions from blood (Phase I)[edit]

- Biological approach for removing the HIV virions from the blood.
- Chemical approach for removing the HIV virions from the blood.
- Physical approach for removing the HIV virions from the blood.

Approaches to catching the virion (Phase I-III, VI, VII)[edit]

- Phagocytosis of the HIV virions.
- Chemical or organic based capture (creation of any skin or additional membrane around the virion) of HIV virions
- Chemical or organic attachments to the virion

Approaches to destroying or damaging the virion or its parts (Phase I-VII)[edit]

Here, "damage" means inhibiting or stopping the ability of virion to process any of the *Phase II-VII*. Here are the different classification of methods:

- By nature of method:
  - Physical methods (*Phase I-VII*)
  - Chemical and biological methods (*Phase I-VII*)

- By damaging target of the HIV virion structure:[30][31]
  - Damaging the Docking Glycoprotein gp120[32] (*Phase I-III, VI, VII*)
  - Damaging the Transmembrane Glycoprotein gp41[33] (*Phase I-III, VI, VII*)
  - Damaging the virion matrix (*Phase I-III, VI, VII*)
  - Damaging the virion Capsid (*Phase I-III, VI, VII*)
  - Damaging the Reverse Transcriptase (*Phase I-VII*)
  - Damaging the RNA (*Phase I-VII*)

Blocking the replication (Phase I)[edit]

- Insertion into blood chemical or organic compounds which binds to the gp120. Hypothetically, it can be pieces of the CD4 cell membranes with receptors. Any chemical and organic alternative (with ability to bind the gp120) of this receptors also can be used.
- Insertion into blood chemical or organic compounds which binds to the receptors of the CD4 cells.

Inhibiting process of phases (drugs already used for this approach)[edit]

- Biological, chemical or physical approach to inhibit the *Attachment*
- Biological, chemical or physical approach to inhibit the *Penetration*
- Biological, chemical or physical approach to inhibit the *Uncoating*
- Biological, chemical or physical approach to inhibit the *Integration*
- Biological, chemical or physical approach to inhibit the *Replication* including introducing a mutation into the HIV
- Biological, chemical or physical approach to inhibit the *Assembling*
- Biological, chemical or physical approach to inhibit (capping) the *Releasing*

Inhibiting the functionality of infected cells (*Phase VI-VII*)[edit]

Inhibiting the life functions of infected cells:

- Inhibiting the metabolism of infected cells
- Inhibiting the energy exchange of infected cells

Future work[edit]

According to Gary J. Nabel of the Vaccine Research Center, NIH, in Bethesda, Maryland, several hurdles must be overcome before scientific research will culminate in a definitive AIDS vaccine.[34] First, greater translation between animal models and human trials must be established. Second, new, more effective, and more easily produced vectors must be identified. Finally, and most importantly, there must arise a robust understanding of the immune response to potential vaccine candidates. Emerging technologies that enable the identification of T-cell-receptor specificities and cytokine profiles will prove valuable in hastening this process. In July 2012 a science group speculated that that an effective vaccine for HIV would be completed in 2019.[35]

A killed whole HIV vaccine, SAV001, that has had success in the US FDA phase 1 human clinical trial in Sep. 2013. This HIV vaccine uses a "dead" version of HIV-1 for the first time. The outcome of the phase 1 human clinical trial has turned out that the vaccine has shown no serious adverse effects while boosting HIV-1 specific antibody. According to Dr. Chil-Yong Kang, the developer of this vaccine, the antibody against gp120 surface antigen and p24 capsid anigen increased to 8-fold and 64-fold, respectively after vaccination.[36]

There have been reports that HIV patients coinfected with GBV-C can survive longer than those without GBV-C, but the patients may be different in other ways. There is current active research into the virus' effects on the immune system in patients coinfected with GBV-C and HIV.

Prophylactic drug[edit]

On July 16, 2012, The Food and Drug Administration approved the first drug shown to reduce the risk of HIV infection. The agency approved Gilead Sciences' pill Truvada as a preventive measure for people who are at high risk of getting HIV through sexual activity.[37]

See also[edit]

- HIV Vaccine Trials Network
- World AIDS Vaccine Day

References[edit]

1. **Jump up** ^ Healy, Melissa (25 April 2013). "Government shuts down AIDS vaccine trial - latimes.com". *Los Angeles Times* (Los Angeles: Tribune Co). ISSN 0458-3035. Retrieved 25 April 2013.
2. ^ Jump up to: *a b* Joint United Nations Programme on HIV/AIDS (UNAIDS) (December 2005). "AIDS epidemic update" (PDF). World Health Organization. Retrieved 2014-04-22.
3. **Jump up** ^ UNAIDS (2004) Report on the global AIDS epidemic, July 2004
4. **Jump up** ^ Shilts, Randy (1987). *And the Band Played On: Politics, People, and the AIDS Epidemic.* (2007 ed.). St. Martin's Press. ISBN 0-312-24135-6. p. 451
5. **Jump up** ^ Watkins DI (Mar 2008). "Basic HIV Vaccine Development". *Top HIV Med* **16** (1): 7–8. ISSN 1542-8826. PMID 18441377.
6. **Jump up** ^ A. S. Fauci, 1996, An HIV vaccine: breaking the paradigms, Proc. Am. Assoc. Phys. 108:6.
7. ^ Jump up to: *a b* Kim D, Elizaga M, Duerr A (March 2007). "HIV vaccine efficacy trials: towards the future of HIV prevention". *Infect. Dis. Clin. North Am.* **21** (1): 201–17, x. doi:10.1016/j.idc.2007.01.006. ISSN 0891-5520. PMID 17502236.
8. ^ Jump up to: *a b* Watkins DI (March 2008). "The hope for an HIV vaccine based on induction of CD8+ T lymphocytes - A Review". *Mem. Inst. Oswaldo Cruz* **103** (2): 119–29. doi:10.1590/S0074-02762008000200001. ISSN 0074-0276. PMC 2997999. PMID 18425263.

9.   **Jump up** ^ Létourneau S, Im EJ, Mashishi T et al. (Oct 2007). "Design and Pre-Clinical Evaluation of a Universal HIV-1 Vaccine". In Nixon, Douglas. *PLoS ONE* **2** (10): e984. doi:10.1371/journal.pone.0000984. PMC 1991584. PMID 17912361.
10.   **Jump up** ^ Poignard P, Sabbe R, Picchio GR et al. (April 1999). "Neutralizing antibodies have limited effects on the control of established HIV-1 infection in vivo". *Immunity* **10** (4): 431–8. doi:10.1016/S1074-7613(00)80043-6. ISSN 1074-7613. PMID 10229186.
11.   **Jump up** ^ Berman PW, Gregory TJ, Riddle L et al. (June 1990). "Protection of chimpanzees from infection by HIV-1 after vaccination with recombinant glycoprotein gp120 but not gp160". *Nature* **345** (6276): 622–5. doi:10.1038/345622a0. ISSN 0028-0836. PMID 2190095.
12.   **Jump up** ^ Connor RI, Korber BT, Graham BS et al. (February 1998). "Immunological and Virological Analyses of Persons Infected by Human Immunodeficiency Virus Type 1 while Participating in Trials of Recombinant gp120 Subunit Vaccines". *Journal of Virology* **72** (2): 1552–76. ISSN 0022-538X. PMC 124637. PMID 9445059.
13.   **Jump up** ^ Morgan C, Marthas M, Miller C et al. (August 2008). "The Use of Nonhuman Primate Models in HIV Vaccine Development". *PLoS Med.* **5** (8): e173. doi:10.1371/journal.pmed.0050173. ISSN 1549-1277. PMC 2504486. PMID 18700814.
14.   **Jump up** ^ Marques, R.; Williams, A.; Eksmond, U.; Wullaert, A.; Killeen, N.; Pasparakis, M.; Kioussis, D.; Kassiotis, G. (2009). "Generalized immune activation as a direct result of activated CD4+ T cell killing". *Journal of Biology* **8** (10): 93. doi:10.1186/jbiol194. PMC 2790834. PMID 19943952. edit
15.   **Jump up** ^ Vrisekoop, N.; Mandl, J. N.; Germain, R. N. (2009). "Life and death as a T lymphocyte: from immune protection to HIV pathogenesis". *Journal of Biology* **8** (10): 91. doi:10.1186/jbiol198. PMC 2790836. PMID 19951397. edit
16.   **Jump up** ^ "New Vaccine Could Turn HIV Into Minor Infection". *Fox News*. 2011-09-29. Retrieved 29 September 2011.
17.   **Jump up** ^ "STEP Study Locations". Retrieved 2008-11-04.
18.   **Jump up** ^ Efficacy Results from the STEP Study (Merck V520 Protocol 023/HVTN 502): A Phase II Test-of-Concept Trial of the MRKAd5 HIV-1 Gag/Pol/Nef Trivalent Vaccine
19.   **Jump up** ^ Sekaly, R. P. (2008). The failed HIV Merck vaccine study: a step back or a launching point for furture vaccine development? Journaly of Cell Biology, 205, (1), 7-12
20.   **Jump up** ^ Timberg, Craig (2007-10-25). "AIDS vaccine may have raised risk of infection". The Washington Post. Retrieved 2007-11-12.

21.   **Jump up** ^ Sekaly RP (January 2008). "The failed HIV Merck vaccine study: a step back or a launching point for future vaccine development?". *J. Exp. Med.* **205** (1): 7–12. doi:10.1084/jem.20072681. ISSN 0022-1007. PMC 2234358. PMID 18195078.

22.   **Jump up** ^ Song, Kyung M.; Ostrom, Carol M. (2007-11-08). "Failure of AIDS vaccine punctures soaring hopes". Seattle Times. Retrieved 2008-10-29.

23.   **Jump up** ^ Iaccino E, Schiavone M, Fiume G, Quinto I, Scala G (Jul 2008). "The aftermath of the Merck's HIV vaccine trial". *Retrovirology* **5**: 56. doi:10.1186/1742-4690-5-56. PMC 2483718. PMID 18597681.

24.   ^ Jump up to: [a] [b] Harmon, Katherine (16 November 2009). "Renewed Hope". *Scientific American* **302** (1) (January 2010). pp. 15–16. doi:10.1038/scientificamerican0110-15. Retrieved 23 December 2009.

25.   **Jump up** ^ Rerks-Ngarm S, Pitisuttithum P, Nitayaphan S et al. (November 2009). "Vaccination with ALVAC and AIDSVAX to Prevent HIV-1 Infection in Thailand". *NEJM* **361** (23): 2209–2220. doi:10.1056/NEJMoa0908492. PMID 19843557.

26.   **Jump up** ^ Ewen Callaway (16 September 2011). "Clues emerge to explain first successful HIV vaccine trial".

27.   **Jump up** ^ "Investing to End the AIDS Epidemic: A new Era for HIV Prevention Research and Development". Retrieved 2010-12-13.

28.   **Jump up** ^ "SSRN-Advanced Purchase Commitments for a Malaria Vaccine: Estimating Costs and Effectiveness by Ernst Berndt, Rachel Glennerster, Michael Kremer, Jean Lee, Ruth Levine, Georg Weizsacker, Heidi Williams". Retrieved 2009-01-10.

29.   **Jump up** ^ Collier, Leslie; Balows, Albert; Sussman, Max (1998) Topley and Wilson's Microbiology and Microbial Infections ninth edition, Volume 1, Virology, volume editors: Mahy, Brian and Collier, Leslie. Arnold. ISBN 0-340-66316-2., 75–91

30.   **Jump up** ^ McGovern SL, Caselli E, Grigorieff N, Shoichet BK (2002). "A common mechanism underlying promiscuous inhibitors from virtual and high-throughput screening". J Med Chem 45 (8): 1712–22. doi:10.1021/jm010533y. PMID 11931626.

31.   **Jump up** ^ Compared with overview in: Fisher, Bruce; Harvey, Richard P.; Champe, Pamela C. (2007). Lippincott's Illustrated Reviews: Microbiology (Lippincott's Illustrated Reviews Series). Hagerstown, MD: Lippincott Williams & Wilkins. ISBN 0-7817-8215-5. Page 3

32.   **Jump up** ^ Kuiken, C., Leitner, T., Foley, B., et al. (2008). "HIV Sequence Compendium", Los Alamos National Laboratory.

33.   **Jump up** ^ Kim PS, Malashkevich VN, Chan DC, Chutkowski CT (1998). "Crystal structure of the simian

immunodeficiency virus (SIV) gp41 core: conserved helical interactions underlie the broad inhibitory activity of gp41 peptides". Proc. Natl. Acad. Sci. U.S.A. 95 (16): 9134-9139. PMID 9689046

34.   **Jump up** ^ Nabel, G. J. (2001). "Challenges and opportunities for development of an AIDS vaccine". *Nature* **410** (6831): 1002–1007. doi:10.1038/35073500. PMID 11309631..

35.   **Jump up** ^ "Scientists see AIDS vaccine within reach after decades | Reuters". *reuters.com*. 2012. Retrieved 17 July 2012.

36.   **Jump up** ^ "New HIV Vaccine Proves Successful In Phase 1 Human Trial". *Medical Daily* (New York). 2013-09-04. Retrieved 2013-09-04.

37.   **Jump up** ^ Perrone, Matthew. "FDA approves first pill to help prevent HIV". *Today Health*. NBC News. Retrieved 16 July 2012.

External links[edit]

- Vaccine Research Center (VRC)- Information concerning Preventive HIV vaccine research studies
- NIAID HIV vaccine site (DAIDS)
- Global Alliance for Vaccines and Immunization (GAVI)
- International AIDS Vaccine Initiative (IAVI)
- AIDS Vaccine Advocacy Coalition (AVAC)
- U.S. Military HIV Research Program (MHRP)
- The Pipeline Project - Vaccines in Development (Center for HIV Information at the University of California San Francisco and the HIV Vaccine Trials Network)
- Capital Area Vaccine Effort CAVE
- Investigation of first candidate vaccine
- Vaccines for Development
- Be the Generation - Information on HIV Vaccine Clinical Research in 20 American Cities
- Australian recruiter for HIV treatment studies
- Aids Vaccine Integrated Project *(European Union research programme)*
- AIDS.gov - The U.S. Federal Domestic HIV/AIDS Resource
- HIVtest.org - Find an HIV testing site near you
- [1]
- - HIV vaccine 'reduces infection'

•

.

www.ingramcontent.com/pod-product-compliance
Lightning Source LLC
Chambersburg PA
CBHW051702170526
45167CB00002B/506